THE ACID REFLUX COOKBOOK

LINDSEY RUSH

Copyright

Plan your journey with
ACID REFLUX

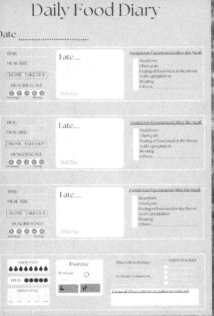

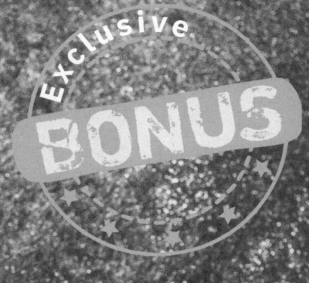

Unique

DAILY FOOD DIARY and much MORE

Use the QR code at the book's last page to access your

SPECIAL BONUSES

Table of Contents

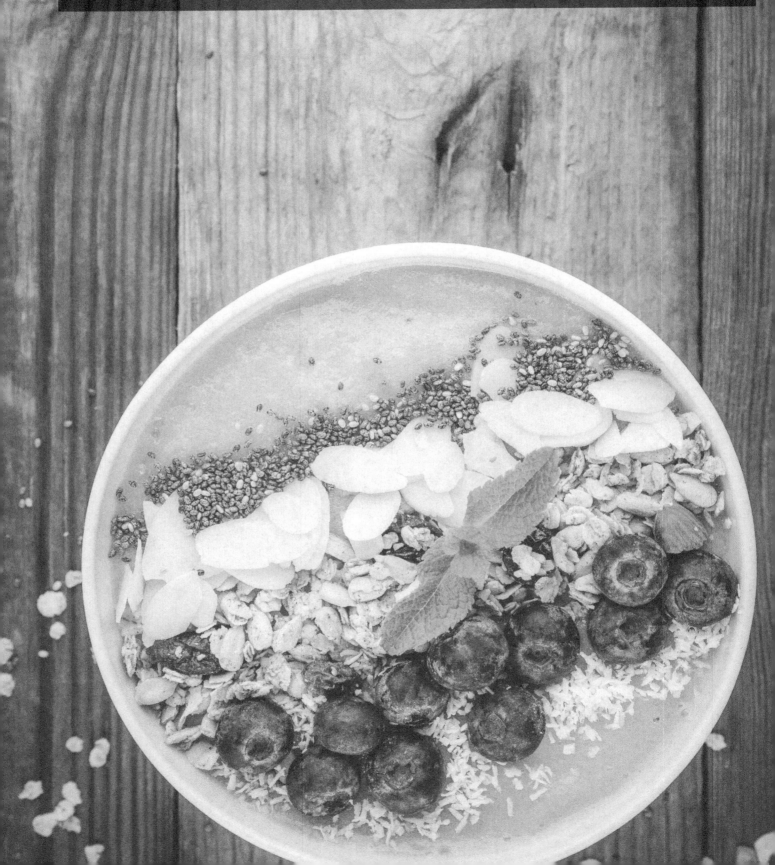

INTRODUCTION..10
Causes of Acid Reflux...11
Symptoms of Acid Reflux...12

CHAPTER 1
FOODS TO AVOID, FOODS TO EAT, AND WHAT TO DRINK............14
Foods to Avoid...15
Foods to Enjoy...15
Dietary and Lifestyle Changes to Soothe Acid Reflux.................16
Stocking Your Pantry and Kitchen...17
Kitchen Tools..17

CHAPTER 2
BREAKFAST...18
1. Steel Cut Oatmeal...19
2. Pine Nut Pesto with Basil..19
3. Broccoli and Squash Mix...20
4. Transition Breakfast Muesli...20
5. Alkaline Fiber Muesli...21
6. Banana Date Porridge..21
7. Blueberry Banana Baked Oatmeal......................................22
8. Seedy Breakfast...23
9. Pistachio and Pecan Granola...23
10. Walnuts Granola for Breakfast..24
11. Watermelon Salad...24
12. Baked Apples with Ginger...25
13. Coconut Porridge..25

CHAPTER 3
SNACKS...27
14. Zucchini Hummus..28
15. Salmon Canapés...28
16. Sweet Potato Fries..29

17. Nuts and Seeds Mix..30
18. Crispy Baked Kale Chips...31
19. Roasted Vegetables..32
20. Crispy Roasted Cauliflower..33
21. Curry-Spiced Nut Mix With Maple Syrup.....................34
22. Baked Herb Zucchini Chips..35
23. Sweet Potato and Celery Root Mash...........................36
24. Kale Chips..36
25. Spiced Nuts...37
26. Homemade Guacamole..37

CHAPTER 4
SOUPS/SALADS

SOUPS/SALADS...39
27. Cabbage and Almond Salad.......................................40
28. Healthy Fruit Salad with Yogurt Cream.......................40
29. Cabbage and Scallions Salad.....................................41
30. Summertime Fruit Salad..42
31. Cranberry Salad...42
32. Tuna and Vegetable Salad...43
33. Chopped Greek Salad..44
34. Cucumber Soup..45
35. Smoked Turkey Salad...45
36. Pork Salad...46
37. Veggie Lunch Salad..47
38. Carrot Cucumber Salad...48
39. Cauliflower Soup..49
40. Purple Potato Soup...50
41. Broccoli Soup..51
42. Leeks Soup..51
43. Mesmerizing Lentil Soup..52
44. Cream of Mushroom Soup...53
45. Roasted Vegetable Soup...54
46. Quick Spinach Salad...54
47. Root Vegetable Salad with Maple Syrup Dressing........55
48. Mackerel Soup...56

49. Kale Soup...56
50. Eggplant Salad...57

CHAPTER 5
LUNCH/DINNER

LUNCH/DINNER..59
51. Chicken with Parsley Sauce.......................................60
52. Chicken and Lentil Casserole....................................61
53. Herb Lamb..62
54. Split Pea Soup with Coconut....................................63
55. Balsamic Scallops..64
56. Coconut Zucchini Cream...64
57. Tender Coconut Chicken...65
58. Vegetarian Pizza with Autumn Toppings....................66
59. Tender Stir-Fry Chicken...67
60. Tuna Stew..67
61. Thyme Chard-Turkey Burgers...................................68
62. Easy Turkey Meatloaf..69
63. Rosemary Broiled Shrimp..69
64. Chicken and Pumpkin Stew.....................................70
65. Turkey Stew...71
66. Pork Chops and Sauce...72
67. Seafood Noodles..73
68. Duck with Bok Choy...74
69. Deliciously Simple Beef...75
70. Holiday Feast Lamb Shanks.....................................76
71. Beef Steaks with Creamy Bacon and Mushrooms........77
72. Cilantro Beef Curry with Cauliflower.........................78
73. Cranberry Pork BBQ Dish...79

CHAPTER 6
SMOOTHIES

SMOOTHIES..81
74. Green Smoothie..82
75. Avocado Smoothie..83
76. Sunshine Smoothie...83

77. Pear and Green Tea Smoothie...84

78. Refreshing Apple Smoothie..85

79. Delicious Mango Smoothie...86

80. Raspberry and Chard Smoothie...86

81. Apple and Kale Smoothie..87

82. Banana Alkaline Smoothie...87

83. Vegetables Smoothie..88

84. Green Apple Smoothie..88

85. Cherry Smoothie...89

86. Mango-Thyme Smoothie..90

87. Peanut Blackberry Smoothie..91

88. Healthy Spinach Smoothie...91

CHAPTER 7
DESSERT

DESSERT...93

89. Strawberry Thumbprint Cookies...94

90. Sweet Banana Pudding...95

91. Grapefruit Sorbet...96

92. Zesty Shortbread Cookies...97

93. Grape Skillet Galette...98

94. Baked Apples with Tahini Raisin Filling...................................99

95. Pistachio and Fruits...100

CHAPTER 8
VEGAN AND VEGETARIAN RECIPES

VEGAN AND VEGETARIAN RECIPES...101

96. Roasted Broccoli and Cashews..102

97. Sweet Potatoes and Pea Hash...103

98. Veggie Kabobs..104

99. Three Beans Chili..105

100. Enjoyable Green Lettuce and Bean Medley.............................106

101. Basil Zucchini Spaghetti...107

102. Healthy, Blistered Beans and Almonds..................................108

CHAPTER 9
28-DAY MEAL PLAN..109

CHAPTER 10
SHOPPING LIST + COOKING CONVERSION CHART...111
Measurement Conversions...112

CONCLUSION..114

Introduction

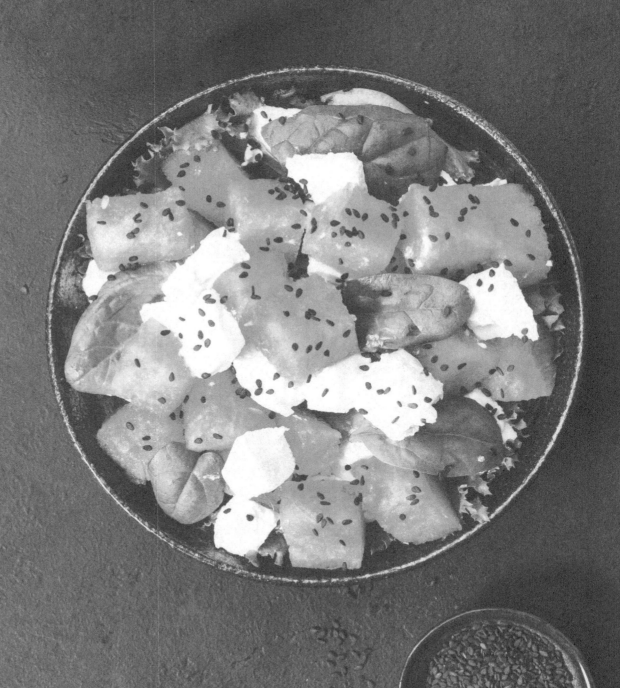

Acid reflux is characterized by a burning pain in the lower chest, food pipe, or throat, similar to heartburn. When stomach acid rises to the food pipe, it causes an acidic sensation in the pipe and lower chest. In severe cases, it can reach the throat, causing severe pain and discomfort. Acid reflux is a common digestive disorder that causes irritation, heartburn, pain at the stomach's opening, and burning in the food canal. This problem is caused by the reverse flow of fluid and food from the stomach to the throat. People all over the world suffer from acid reflux and other related issues, which can worsen if not treated promptly and properly.

A person's productivity and thinking ability can suffer as a result of ongoing gastric issues. It can limit a person's activities and be the source of a severe ulcer or esophageal cancer. A lifestyle change is the most effective and natural way to treat acid reflux and its complications. Following proper diet plans and implementing exercise routines can aid in the treatment of reflux and improve digestive health. Acid reflux can easily affect people who are obese, diabetic or have inflammation issues.

This book will go over foods that can help you control acid reflux as well as foods to avoid if you want to keep these symptoms at bay. This book contains not only information about acid reflux but also recipes and a 28-day meal plan. The most difficult aspect of making a lifestyle change is getting started. I wanted to make the process a little easier by providing you with the information you need to get started. You can get started right away without having to do a lot of planning.

This book is not intended to be a fact sheet or a recipe book but rather a lifestyle guide. You should leave fully equipped with the knowledge you need to start living a healthier lifestyle. As a result, we can't just dive into the how-tos. You must understand what acid reflux is, what causes it, and how to manage it. It's similar to laying a foundation.

Causes of Acid Reflux

Acid reflux occurs when some of your stomach's acidity flows into your esophagus or gullet. Heartburn, despite its name, has nothing to do with the heart. The stomach contains hydrochloric acid, a strong acid that aids digestion while also protecting against infections such as germs. The stomach lining is specially designed to protect the stomach from a strong acid, but the esophagus is not. The gastroesophageal sphincter is a muscular ring that acts as a valve, allowing food to enter the stomach but not return to the esophagus. When this valve fails and stomach contents regurgitate into the esophagus, acid reflux symptoms such as heartburn occur.

Obesity is another cause of gastric acid reflux. When we do not manage our weight, our bodies behave differently. Above-average weight causes a strong reaction in the body. Organs begin to behave abnormally, which can cause problems. Obesity is not normal; it is associated with some health risks. Weight and mass gain have an impact on total body stamina, bone strength, heart performance, blood circulation, hormonal changes, and organ activity.

One of the significant consequences of obesity is gastric acid reflux. The stomach cannot properly digest all of the food, and the acid release is an attempt to deal with the excess energy in the body. It causes the stomach acid to flow outward. Furthermore, obesity can affect stomach size, and its movement can cause acid reflux.

Smoking also has an impact on the overall organ system composition. It can harm not only the lungs but also the stomach. In response to the smoke and all of its chemicals, the acid in the stomach travels back to the food canal. When a person inhales and exhales smoke, acid fumes from the stomach can escape, increasing the risks and effects of gastric acid reflux.

Alcoholism is hazardous to one's overall health. It has an impact on one's lifestyle as well as the body's internal organs. Alcohol consumption is beneficial when kept within a safe limit, but when it is excessive, problems arise. Acid reflux is one of the issues that can arise from excessive alcohol consumption. The important thing is to keep alcohol consumption routine and limited for safe use.

Acid reflux can occur when a person eats and engages in no or little physical activity. The stomach produces acid to digest food, but too much acid causes reflux in the food canal when there is no activity. It is critical to walk after a meal or physically exert your body in order to trigger proper digestion of your food. It will assist you in making things better and smoother. Physical activity will help you use the acid in your stomach more effectively and dissolve it in your food. It will neutralize the acid in the digestive process and provide you with all of the nutrients you require. Our sedative and antidepressant medications can occasionally cause stomach acidity. This acidity can eventually cause gastric acid reflux.

Several changes occur during pregnancy. Everything changes, from mood swings to food choices, and psychological concepts to physical movements. Females face numerous threats during this process, many of which are critical health constraints. It can happen as a result of a lack of care, vitamins, or overuse of a specific product. There are also genetic reactions in the body on occasion. Acid reflux is not inherited, but it can be triggered by pregnancy and hormonal changes. Your stomach may act differently, and you may not get as much physical movement, resulting in reflux.

Furthermore, the vomiting and nausea caused by pregnancy can always cause gastric acid reflux. The important thing in this regard is to monitor everything and then have essential solutions.

When it comes to your overall health, your food intake and dietary choices are extremely important. Acid reflux can be triggered by poor dietary choices. If you consume junk food, soft drinks, dried snacks, and fat-rich foods, you may develop acid reflux. Such foods increase stomach acidity, which can lead to problems.

Acid reflux is caused by more than just medical deficiencies and complications. It may appear as a result of poor posture. When eating, it is critical to maintain proper physical posture. Acid reflux can be caused by bending over your waist or lying on your back while eating or immediately after eating.

It can be dangerous and build up the issue for more serious causes. It is necessary to watch out during your meal and pay attention to your movement routine to avoid such drastic outcomes from your activities.

Symptoms of Acid Reflux

One of the most common symptoms of acid reflux is heartburn. It is not the same thing, but it is the first step toward the condition. You may experience discomfort or pain in your abdomen and chest area, which extends up to your throat.

Another sign of bad stomach conditions and acid reflux is a bitter taste in the back of the mouth and throat.

The sensation of nausea or the desire to vomit after eating.

Constant burping with a foul odor and an acidic sensation.

In severe cases, vomiting can be bloody and painful.

Acid reflux can result in black and bloody stools and a burning sensation.

There may be painful hiccups accompanied by a burning sensation.

The drastic weight loss can be seen for no apparent reason.

In both the acute and chronic stages of acid reflux, sore throat, dry cough, and wheezing can occur.

There may be a feeling of unease in the throat as if food is stuck there.

Difficulty swallowing food, accompanied by a burning sensation.

Bad breath and dental erosion are other major symptoms of acid reflux.

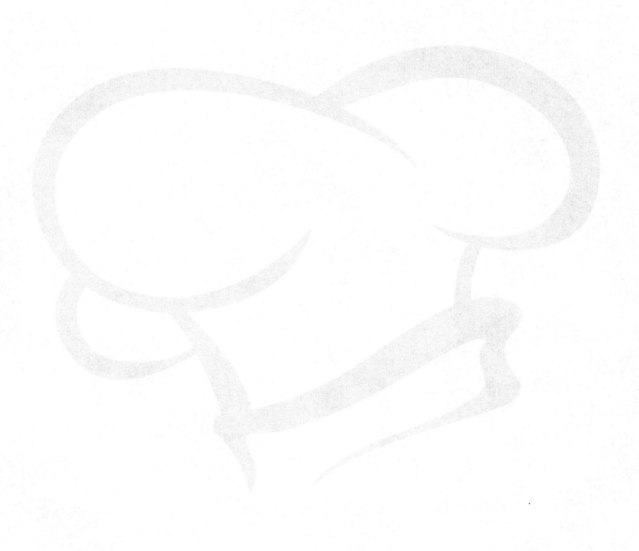

CHAPTER 1
Foods to Avoid, Foods to Eat, and What to Drink

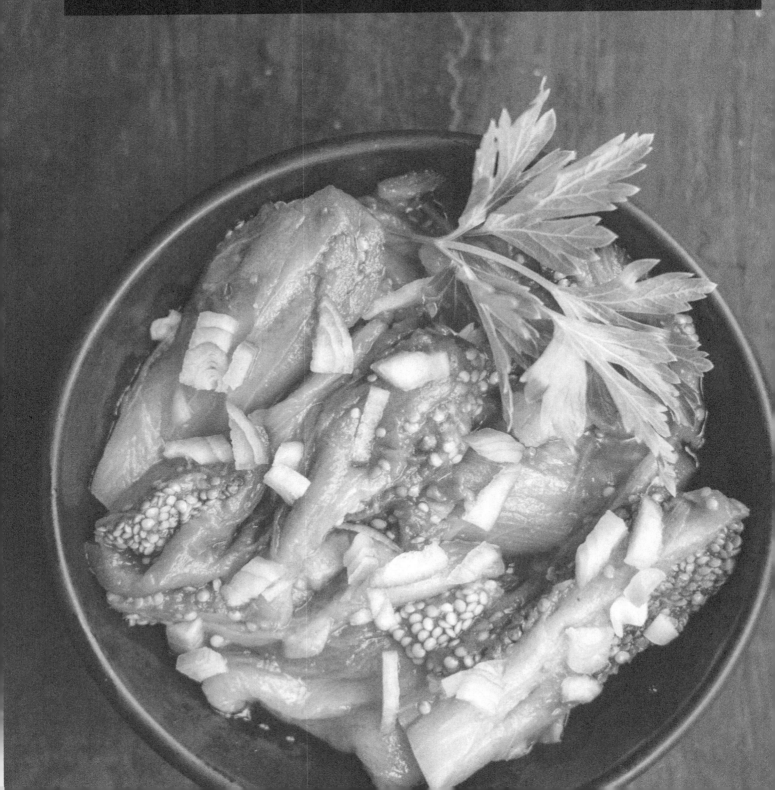

The following are helpful summaries of foods to avoid to improve your symptoms, as well as foods to consume in moderation and foods you can enjoy without worrying they will trigger a flare-up.

Foods to Avoid

- Alcoholic beverages
- Artificial Sweeteners
- Caffeine and mint
- Carbonated beverages
- Chillis, hot sauce
- Chocolate
- Citrus fruits
- Fresh tomato
- Cream sauces
- Dairy
- Fried foods
- Garlic
- Mint teas
- Margarine
- Spicy food

Foods to Enjoy

- Agave nectar
- Apple red
- Avocado
- Banana
- Beef, extra-lean cuts
- Berries
- Bread and muffins
- Celery
- Cereal whole-grain
- Cheese   Nonfat
- Citrus zest
- Corn
- Eggs
- Fennel
- Fish and shellfish
- Fish sauce
- Ginger fresh or ground
- Grains
- Honey
- Legumes

- Maple syrup
- Melon, honeydew, or watermelon
- Miso
- Mushrooms
- Oatmeal
- Olive oil
- Olives
- Pasta
- Pear
- Popcorn
- Poultry skinless, not fried
- Poultry broth or stock
- Rice
- Sea salt
- Soy sauce
- Sugar
- Tofu
- Vegetables
- Yogurt low-fat, plain, nonfat

Dietary and Lifestyle Changes to Soothe Acid Reflux

Midnight acid reflux causes discomfort, and the resulting bitter taste can not only disrupt but also make sleep difficult. Here are some helpful hints to help you do just that:

- **Keep a healthy weight.** Even a slight weight gain can aggravate heartburn symptoms. Maintaining a healthy body weight can help you reduce acid reflux symptoms.
- **Dress comfortably.** Tight clothing, particularly around the waist, can put a strain on the stomach. Acid reflux symptoms may worsen as a result of this. As a result, wear loose-fitting clothing, especially around the waist and when going to bed.
- **Avoid eating trigger foods.** Keep a list of the foods that cause acid reflux. These foods may differ from person to person. Exacerbating foods include onions, garlic, peppermint, caffeinated beverages, chocolate, fatty foods, and spicy or fried foods. Citrus fruits, such as oranges, can also cause acid reflux.
- **Relax and enjoy your meal.** Eating under stress or in a hurry can increase the production of stomach acids. Relax after you've finished your meals. Avoid lying down, however. Choose relaxation techniques such as meditation, yoga, or deep breathing.
- **Avoid late-night eating and large meals.** Make it a point to eat your last meal of the day at least 2 to 3 hours before going to bed. This reduces stomach acid while allowing the stomach to partially empty its contents before sleeping. Large meals can cause stomach discomfort. As a result, instead of three large meals per day, try to eat 5–6 small meals. Also, avoid eating large meals late at night.
- **Maintain your upright position after eating.** Staying upright after eating lowers the risk of stomach acid backing up into the esophagus. Also, after eating, avoid bending over or straining to lift heavy objects.
- **Caffeine consumption should be reduced.** Many people experience acid reflux after drinking coffee, according to research. Most patients report significant relief after reducing their coffee consumption. As a result, you should limit your leisurely cup of coffee for weekend breakfast to avoid acid reflux symptoms.

- **Stop smoking.** The negative health effects of smoking are well known, and they extend into the realm of GERD by increasing stomach acid production and weakening the LES, making you more prone to reflux and other GERD-related symptoms.
- **Eat fewer, smaller meals more frequently.** Because people suffering from GERD and related symptoms frequently have a malfunctioning lower esophageal sphincter, you want to make that muscle's job as simple as possible.
- **Eat for at least four hours before going to bed.** Lying down with a full stomach does two things: it increases IAP and puts you in a position that allows stomach contents to move easily upward through the LES. Give your food time to digest. Stop eating four hours before bedtime and you'll be less likely to have nighttime GERD symptoms.

Stocking Your Pantry and Kitchen

For optimal health and GERD management, a high-fiber, plant-based diet is usually the best way to go. These principles are emphasized by the pantry essentials I've chosen. Whenever possible, I provide substitutes for common trigger foods and consider FODMAPs for those who may be affected by them. Here are a few ingredients to keep on hand:

- Almonds, chopped
- Chia seeds
- Cinnamon
- Cumin
- Ginger, ground
- Honey
- Maple syrup, pure
- Olive oil (and olive oil cooking spray)
- Sea salt
- Low-sodium soy sauce
- Thyme, dried

Kitchen Tools

- Various sizes of baking sheets and pans for stovetop grilling
- Food processor and/or blender
- Chopping boards (at least two)
- Airtight storage containers made of glass or plastic
- Set of knives
- Saucepans made of parchment paper of various sizes
- Dutch oven
- Large nonstick skillet
- Slow cooker
- Soup maker
- Steaming basket
- Vegetable peeler
- Wood spoons

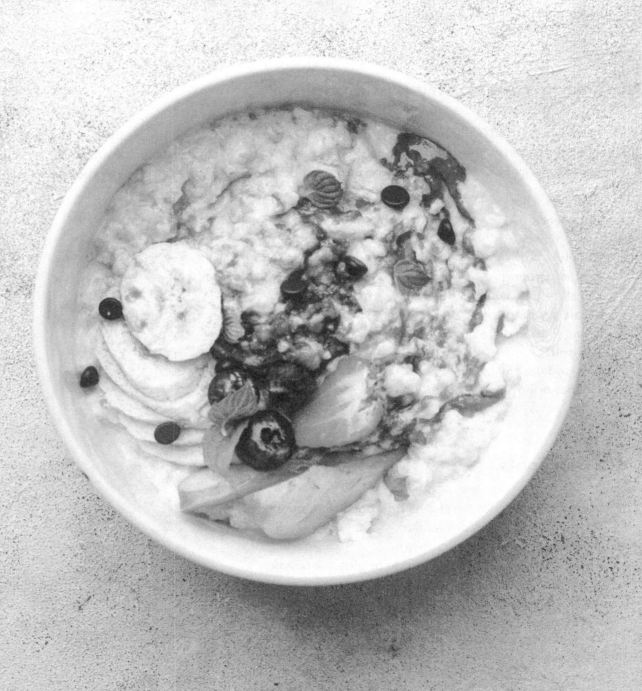

1. Steel Cut Oatmeal

 15 minutes   35 minutes   1

Ingredients

- 1 tbsp almond butter
- 1 cup steel-cut oats
- 3 cups boiling water
- 1/2 cup almond milk
- 1/2 cup plus 1 tbsp cashew milk
- 1 tbsp Splenda

Directions

1. Heat almond butter with oats in a saucepan.
2. Stir cook for 2 minutes, then stirs in boiling water.
3. Bring the mixture to a low simmer and cook for 25 minutes.
4. Add half of the almond and cashew milk and cook for 10 minutes.
5. Stir in all the remaining ingredients.
6. Serve.

Nutrition

Calories: 428, **Fat:** 16.6 g, **Carbs:** 51.4 g, **Protein:** 18.1 g

2. Pine Nut Pesto with Basil

 12 minutes   2 minutes   4

Ingredients

- 3/4 cup extra-virgin olive oil, plus more as needed
- 1/3 cup pine nuts
- 3 cups firmly packed basil leaves
- 1/2 tsp kosher salt

Directions

1. Place a skillet over medium heat and warm it. Stir in the pine nuts, cook, and stir constantly for 2 minutes until they are lightly browned. Place into a plate to cool.
2. In a food processor, add cooled pine nuts. Add the basil and pulse another ten times. Pour in the olive oil slowly with the motor running, and puree until the pesto is the texture of a coarse paste. Stir in more oil or 2 to 3 tbsp water if you like a thinner one. Add salt.
3. Place in an airtight container, top a thin layer of olive oil over, and store in the refrigerator for up to 1 week.

Nutrition

Calories: 400, **Fat:** 42.5 g, **Protein:** 3.3 g, **Carbs:** 0.8 g

3. Broccoli and Squash Mix

10 minutes   15 minutes   4

Ingredients

- 4 cups spaghetti squash, peeled, cooked and flesh scrapped out
- 1 1/2 cups broccoli florets
- 1 tbsp olive oil
- 1 cup coconut milk, unsweetened
- A pinch of salt

Directions

1. Heat a pan with the oil over medium-high heat, and add the spaghetti squash and the broccoli. Stir and cook for 5 to 6 minutes. Add the salt and cook for 5 minutes more. Add the coconut milk, mix, and cook for about 5 minutes more, then divide into bowls and serve for breakfast.
2. Enjoy!

Nutrition

Calories: 204, **Fat:** 16.2g, **Carbs:** 10.4 g, **Protein:** 4.2 g

4. Transition Breakfast Muesli

5 minutes   0 minutes   1

Ingredients

- Handful organic oats
- Handful almonds
- Handful walnuts
- Handful cranberries
- 1 banana
- 1 cup rice milk for taste

Directions

1. Combine the ingredients, then serve with your preferred milk.

Nutrition

Calories: 499, **Fat:** 27.3 g, **Carbs:** 49.7 g, **Protein:** 14.5 g

5. Alkaline Fiber Muesli

 5 minutes 0 minutes 1

Ingredients

- Toasted oats to taste
- A handful of almond meal
- A small handful of psyllium husks
- Handful sliced almonds
- Handful sunflower seeds, sliced
- Handful of buckwheat
- 1/2 apple, grated
- 1 cup almond milk for taste

Directions

1. Mix all ingredients and as much milk as you want to create muesli.

Nutrition

Calories: 497, **Fat:** 31 g, **Carbs:** 35.5 g, **Protein:** 19.1 g

6. Banana Date Porridge

 5 minutes 10 minutes 2

Ingredients

- 1 cup oats
- 2 cups water
- 2 bananas, mashed half and sliced half
- 2 dates, finely chopped
- 2 tsp vanilla bean paste

Directions

1. In a small saucepan, heat the oats and water. Simmer for 5 minutes or until most of the water has been absorbed. While the oats are cooking, chop the date and mash half of the banana. Cook for at least 5 minutes after adding the cinnamon, banana, vanilla, and date to the porridge. Pour into a bowl and top with banana slices.

Nutrition

Calories: 271, **Fat:** 3.1 g, **Carbs:** 55.2 g, **Protein:** 8.6 g

7. Blueberry Banana Baked Oatmeal

5 minutes   55 minutes   8

Ingredients

- 2 cups regular rolled oats
- 2 cups boiling water
- 2 large bananas (+ 1/2 for topping)
- 1 egg
- 1/4 cup hemp seeds
- 1/2 cup blueberries
- 1/4 cup sliced almonds
- 2 tsp cinnamon
- 1 tsp vanilla

Directions

1. In a mixing bowl, combine the oats and boiling water. Allow for 10 to 15 minutes of resting time. Meanwhile, mash the banana until smooth, then stir in the egg. Pour this mixture over the softened oats and mix well. Stir in the remaining ingredients until thoroughly combined. Fill a 9x13 baking pan halfway with the oat mixture. Serve with sliced bananas and blueberries on top. Bake for 55 to 60 minutes at 375°F. Allow cooling slightly before cutting into and serving.

Nutrition

Calories: 134, **Carbs:** 17.5 g, **Protein:** 5.7 g, **Fat:** 4.5 g

8. Seedy Breakfast

5 minutes   0 minutes   8

Ingredients

- 2 cups sunflower seeds with 2 cups pumpkin seed
- 2 cups almonds
- 2 cups sesame seeds with1 apple, grated
- 1 cup alkaline water
- 1oz soy milk

Directions

1. For 3 hours, the seed and apple mixture should be soaked in soy milk and alkaline water.
2. To change the flavor, you can add more soy milk when it's finished. Add the other ingredients.

Nutrition

Calories: 487, **Fat:** 36.1 g, **Carbs:** 24.8 g, **Protein:** 16.5 g

9. Pistachio and Pecan Granola

10 minutes   25 minutes   8

Ingredients

- 2 cups rolled oats
- 1/2 cup chopped pecans
- 1/2 cup shelled pistachios
- 1/4 cup coconut oil, melted
- 1/4 cup honey
- 1/4 tsp sea salt

Directions

1. Preheat oven to 350°F. Line a baking sheet with parchment paper.
2. In a large bowl, combine oats, pecans, and pistachios.
3. In a separate bowl, whisk together coconut oil, honey, and salt.
4. Pour the wet ingredients over the dry ingredients and mix until everything is evenly coated.
5. Spread the granola mixture onto the prepared baking sheet.
6. Bake for 25 minutes, stirring every 10 minutes, until golden brown.
7. Let cool completely before transferring to an airtight container.

Nutrition

Calories: 235, **Protein:** 6 g, **Carbs:** 17.6 g, **Fat:** 15.7 g

10. Walnuts Granola for Breakfast

 10 minutes 20 minutes 8

Ingredients

- 3 cups rolled oats
- 1/2 cup walnuts, chopped
- 1/4 cup honey
- 1/4 cup olive oil
- 1/4 tsp sea salt

Directions

1. Preheat oven to 350°F.
2. In a large bowl, mix together oats, walnuts, honey, olive oil, ginger, turmeric, and salt.
3. Spread the mixture onto a baking sheet lined with parchment paper.
4. Bake for 20 minutes, stirring every 5 minutes, until golden brown.
5. Let cool before serving.

Nutrition

Calories: 227, **Protein:** 6.2 g, **Carbs:** 22.3 g, **Fat:** 12.7 g

11. Watermelon Salad

 10 minutes 0 minutes 2

Ingredients

- 1/2 tsp agave nectar
- 1 tbsp extra-virgin olive oil
- 12 oz watermelon, chopped
- 1/2 cup chopped basil leaves
- 2 cups baby arugula

Directions

1. In a bowl, toss together the watermelon, basil, arugula, oil, and agave nectar. Serve for breakfast.

Nutrition

Calories: 151, **Fat:** 8 g, **Carbs:** 17.7 g, **Protein:** 1.8 g

12. Baked Apples with Ginger

10 minutes   40 minutes   6

Ingredients

- 4 apples
- 2 ginger, chopped
- 4 prunes, chopped
- 3 tbsp muscovado sugar
- 1 tbsp butter

Directions

1. Preheat the oven to 200°F. Cut a quarter of each apple and set them into a baking dish.
2. Take a bowl, add ginger, sugar, prunes, and butter, and mix well. Pour the mixture over the apples and put the butter on each apple's top.
3. Bake them for 35 minutes or until cooked well.
4. Remove and serve the hot baked apple.

Nutrition

Calories: 209, **Fat:** 2.7 g, **Carbs:** 45.1 g, **Protein:** 1.3 g

13. Coconut Porridge

10 minutes   15 minutes   4

Ingredients

- 2 cups coconut milk, unsweetened
- 3 tbsp almond flour
- 1/2 cup coconut flakes, unsweetened
- 2 tbsp ground flax meal
- 1 tsp vanilla extract

Directions

1. In a small pot, mix the coconut milk with the almond flour, coconut flakes, flax meal, and vanilla. Stir and bring to a simmer over medium heat for 15 minutes. Divide into bowls and serve for breakfast.
2. Enjoy!

Nutrition

Calories: 372, **Fat:** 35 g, **Carbs:** 8.1 g, **Protein:** 5.5 g

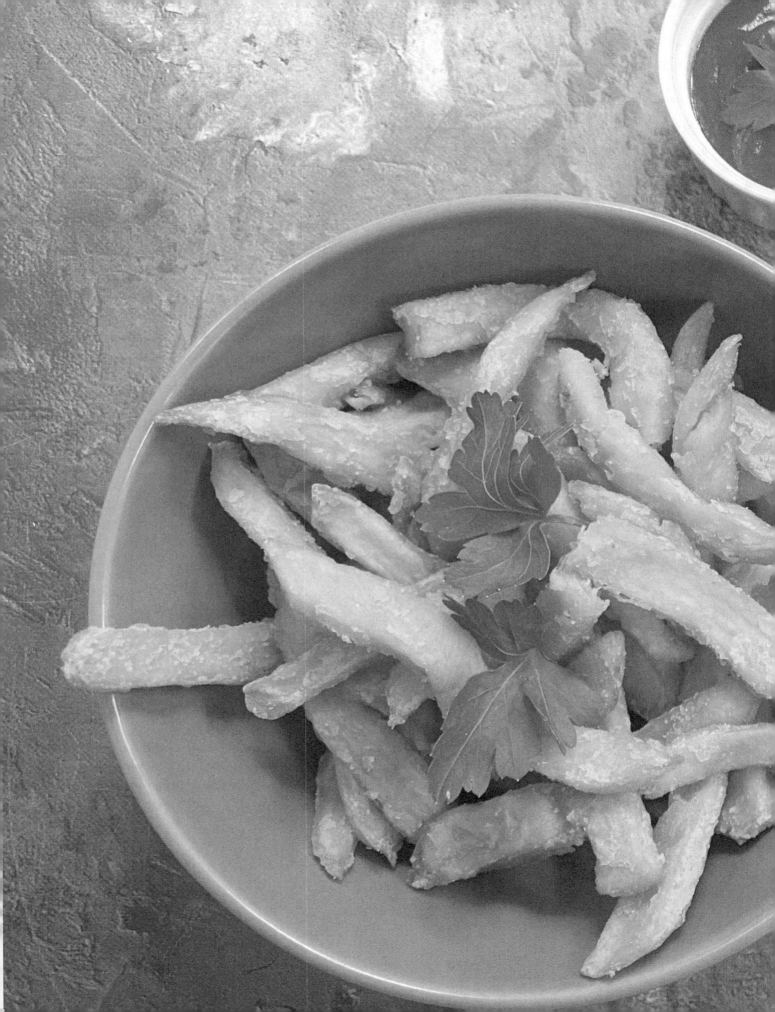

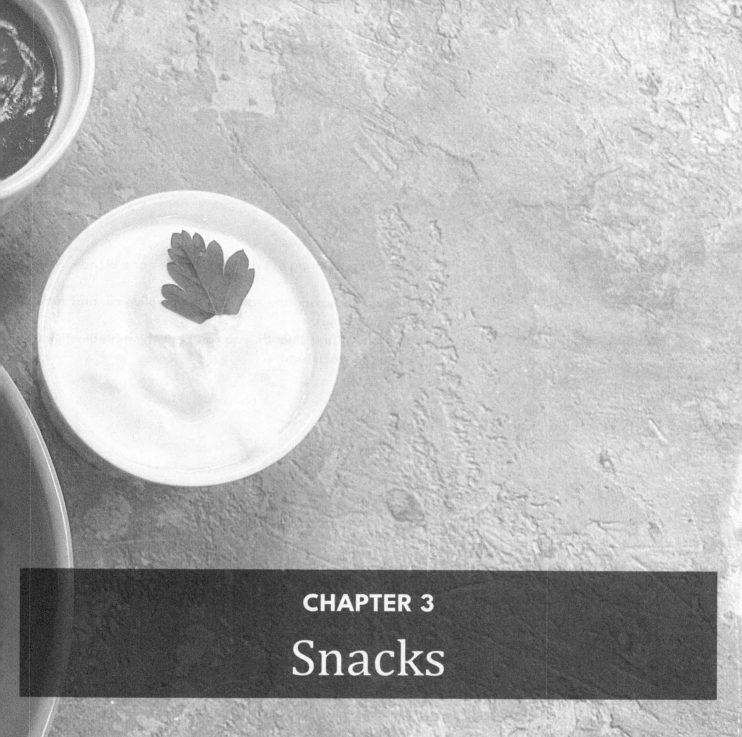

CHAPTER 3
Snacks

14. Zucchini Hummus

15 minutes

2

0 minutes

Ingredients

- 1 tsp salt
- 1 tsp chopped dill, fresh
- 1 tbsp tahini
- 1 tbsp olive oil
- 1 chopped zucchini

Directions

1. To start this recipe, bring out a food processor or a blender and set it up.
2. When that is ready, add the salt, dill, tahini, olive oil, and zucchini to the mix and blend.
3. When this is nice and smooth, you can pour the ingredients into a bowl and serve when ready.

Nutrition

Calories: 130, **Fat:** 11.7 g,, **Carbs:** 3.5 g, **Protein:** 2.7 g

15. Salmon Canapés

20 minutes   0 minutes   2

Ingredients

- 1 sliced zucchini in 12 rounds
- 1 tsp salt
- 1 tsp tarragon chopped
- 1/4 cup plain yogurt
- 4 oz canned salmon

Directions

1. For this recipe, take out a bowl before combining the tarragon, salt, yogurt, and salmon.
2. When this is ready, lay out the zucchini rounds flatly. Add the salmon mixture on top of the zucchini rounds and enjoy it.

Nutrition

Calories: 134, **Fat:** 6.8 g, **Carbs:** 3.9 g, **Protein:** 14.2 g

16. Sweet Potato Fries

15 minutes   25 minutes   1

Ingredients

- 1 sliced sweet potato
- 1 tbsp olive oil
- 1/2 tsp salt
- 1 tsp ground cumin

Directions

1. Turn on the oven and give it time to heat up to 450°F.
2. While the oven is heating up, take out a bowl so you can toss together the olive oil, salt, cumin, and sweet potato sticks.
3. When combined well, you can pour them onto a baking sheet with a rim. Make sure that it is all in a single layer.
4. Add the baking sheet with the ingredients into the oven and let them bake. You will need to keep a spatula on hand to flip these around to cook evenly halfway through the process.
5. After 20 minutes or so, the sweet potato fries should be done. You can take them out of the oven before serving.

Nutrition

Calories: 413, **Fat:** 15.9 g, **Carbs:** 63.9 g, **Protein:** 3.6 g

17. Nuts and Seeds Mix

 10 minutes   0 minutes   12

Ingredients

- 1 cup pecans
- 1 cup hazelnuts
- 1 cup almonds
- 1/4 cup coconut, shredded
- 1 cup walnuts
- 1/2 cup papaya pieces, dried
- 1/2 cup dates, dried, pitted, and chopped
- 1/2 cup sunflower seeds
- 1/2 cup pumpkin seeds
- 1 cup raisins

Directions

1. In a bowl, combine the pecans with all the hazelnuts, almonds, coconut, walnuts, papaya, dates, sunflower seeds, pumpkin seeds, and raisins, toss and serve as a snack.
2. Enjoy!

Nutrition

Calories: 370, **Fat:** 29.3 g, **Carbs:** 19.2 g, **Protein:** 45 g

18. Crispy Baked Kale Chips

 15 minutes   14–16   3

minutes

Ingredients

- 1 to 2 tbsp olive oil
- 1 bunch Lacinato kale, rinsed, thoroughly dried, and stems removed
- 1/4 tsp sea salt

Directions

1. Preheat the oven to 350°F.
2. Cut into 2-in (5-cm) pieces of kale leaves, and transfer them to a large bowl. Add the salt and 1 tbsp olive oil. Use your fingers to rub the leaves, and let them coat well with the oil, adding up to another 1 tbsp if needed. Transfer the kale onto two baking sheets, be sure that there is about 1 in (2.5 cm) between the leaves. The leaves will steam instead of crisping if they're too close.
3. Bake for 8 minutes. Take out from the oven and toss the leaves, then return and bake another 6 to 8 minutes until the leaves are crisp. Allow cool.
4. Place in an airtight container, and store at room temperature for up to 1 week.

Nutrition

Calories: 106, **Fat:** 10.2 g, **Protein:** 2.3 g, **Carbs:** 1.3 g

19. Roasted Vegetables

10 minutes   52 minutes   8

Ingredients

- 1 small butternut squash (cubed)
- 2 small Yukon Gold potatoes (cubed)
- 2 medium zucchinis (diced)
- 1 small sweet potato (peeled and cubed)
- 1 tbsp fresh thyme (chopped)
- 3 tbsp olive oil
- 2 tbsp fresh rosemary (chopped)
- 1 1/2 tbsp balsamic vinegar
- 1 tsp salt to taste

Directions

1. Preheat the oven to 475°F. Combine the squash, sweet potato, zucchini, and Yukon Gold potatoes in a large mixing basin. Combine the thyme, rosemary, vinegar, olive oil, and salt in a small bowl. Toss the veggies in the oil mixture until they are well covered. In a big pan, spread evenly. Roast for 30–40 minutes, tossing every 10 minutes, or until veggies are cooked and browned in the oven.

Nutrition

Calories: 163, **Carbs:** 21.1 g, **Protein:** 4.4 g, **Fat:** 6.8 g

20. Crispy Roasted Cauliflower

10 minutes   15 minutes   2

Ingredients

- 1 1/2 tsp ground cumin
- 1 tsp salt
- 1 head cauliflower, roughly chopped into bite-size pieces
- 3 tbsp coconut oil melted

Directions

1. Preheat the oven to 450°F.
2. Combine the cumin and salt in a bowl.
3. Spread the cauliflower in a baking pan, and drizzle with the coconut oil. Sprinkle with the spice mixture and toss to coat.
4. Bake for about 15 minutes.

Nutrition

Calories: 238, **Fat:** 23.2 g, **Protein:** 3.6 g, **Carbs:** 3.5 g

21. Curry-Spiced Nut Mix With Maple Syrup

10 minutes   30–35   6

minutes

Ingredients

- 1/2 cup raw pumpkin seeds
- 1/2 cup raw macadamia nuts, roughly chopped
- 1 cup raw cashew pieces
- 2 tsp maple syrup
- 1 tbsp fresh-pressed coconut oil
- 2 tsp curry powder
- 1/2 tsp kosher salt

Directions

1. Preheat the oven to 300°F. Use parchment paper to line a baking sheet.
2. In a large bowl, add the pumpkin seeds, macadamias, and cashews.
3. Add the maple syrup and coconut oil into a medium saucepan, and melt over low heat for about 1 minute. Remove from the heat and pour over the nut mixture. Add the curry powder, and salt and stir well to coat. Spread the mixture on the prepared baking sheet.
4. Bake for 30 to 35 minutes, until the nuts are light brown, stirring once. Allow cool on the baking sheet.
5. Transfer into an airtight container, and store at room temperature for up to 3 days.

Nutrition

Calories: 278, **Fat:** 20.4 g, **Protein:** 6.6 g, **Carbs:** 17 g

22. Baked Herb Zucchini Chips

15 minutes   2 hours   2

Ingredients

- 2 medium zucchinis, sliced thin with a mandolin or sharp knife
- 1 1/2 tsp dried oregano
- 1 1/2 tsp dried rosemary
- 1 1/2 tsp dried basil
- 2 tbsp extra-virgin olive oil
- 1/2 tsp salt

Directions

1. Preheat the oven to low, usually 175°F to 200°F.
2. Use parchment paper to line two baking sheets.
3. Add the zucchini with the olive oil into a large bowl, and toss together.
4. Add the basil, oregano, rosemary and salt to a small bowl, and stir them together. Place the herbs on top of the zucchini. Mix all the ingredients with your hands to ensure the zucchini is evenly coated.
5. Transfer the zucchini into a single layer on the prepared sheets. They can be close together.
6. Place the sheets in the preheated oven and bake for about 2 hours or until dry and crispy. The baking time depends on your oven's lowest temperature and how thin you cut the zucchini.
7. Allow cooling completely. Store in a sealed container.

Nutrition

Calories: 168, **Fat:** 15.5 g, **Protein:** 2.9 g, **Carbs:** 4.2 g

23. Sweet Potato and Celery Root Mash

5 minutes

20-25 mins

4

Ingredients

- 2 cups chopped sweet potatoes
- 2 cups chopped celery root, scrubbed, trimmed, and peeled
- 2 tbsp almond butter
- 1/2 tsp salt

Directions

1. Place a steamer basket in a large saucepan with 1 to 2 inches of filtered water. Put the sweet potatoes and celery root in the steamer basket.
2. Cover and steam over medium heat for about 20 to 25 minutes until fork-tender.
3. Transfer them to a blender or food processor, along with the almond butter, and sea salt. Blend until completely smooth. Serve immediately.

Nutrition

Calories: 121, **Fat:** 4.3 g, **Protein:** 3.2 g, **Carbs:** 17.6 g

24. Kale Chips

10 minutes

15 minutes

1

Ingredients

- 1 bunch kale leaves
- 1 tbsp organic olive oil

Directions

1. Spread the kale leaves over a baking sheet, add oil and paprika, toss, introduce inside oven, and bake at 350°F for a quarter-hour.
2. Divide into bowls and serve to be a snack.
3. Enjoy!

Nutrition

Calories: 180, **Fat:** 15.1 g, **Carbs:** 3.3 g, **Protein:** 2.7 g

25. Spiced Nuts

 10 minutes 10-15 mins 6

Ingredients

- 1 cup almonds
- 1/2 cup walnuts
- 1/4 cup pumpkin seeds
- 1/4 cup sunflower seeds
- 1/2 tsp ground cumin
- 1 tsp ground turmeric

Directions

1. Preheat the oven to 350°F.
2. In a medium bowl, stir together all the ingredients until well combined.
3. Spread the nuts out onto a rimmed baking sheet and bake for 10 to 15 minutes, stirring once or twice halfway through, or until the nuts are lightly browned and fragrant.
4. Let the nuts cool for 5 to 10 minutes before serving.

Nutrition

Calories: 294, **Fat:** 23.2 g, **Protein:** 9.3 g, **Carbs:** 12.2 g

26. Homemade Guacamole

 10 minutes 0 minutes 4

Ingredients

- 2 ripe avocados, peeled, pitted, and cubed
- 2 tbsp chopped fresh cilantro leaves
- 1/2 tsp sea salt

Directions

1. Place the avocados, cilantro, and sea salt in a medium bowl. Mash them lightly with the back of a fork until a uniform consistency is achieved.
2. Serve chilled.

Nutrition

Calories: 277, **Fat:** 26.8 g, **Protein:** 5.3 g, **Carbs:** 3.4 g

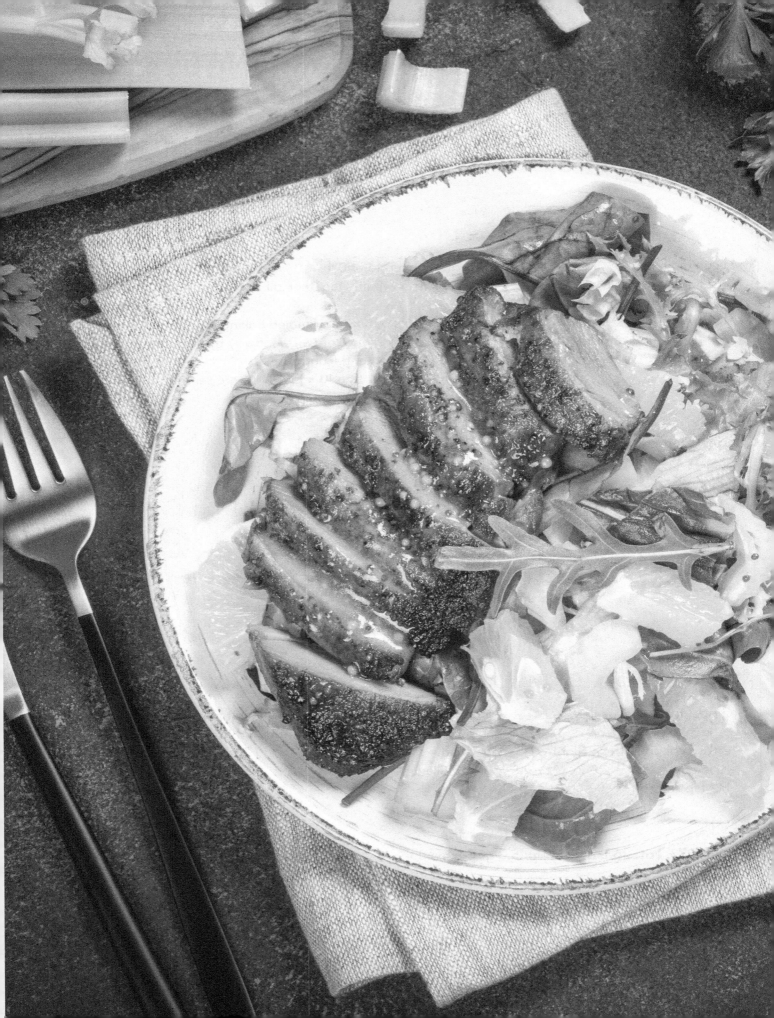

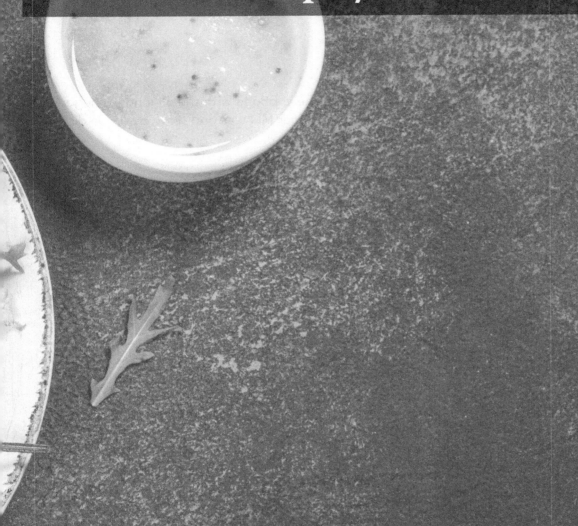

CHAPTER 4
Soups/Salads

27. Cabbage and Almond Salad

10 minutes   0 minutes   4

Ingredients

- 1 Napa cabbage, shredded
- 1 cup chopped almonds
- 1/4 cup balsamic vinegar
- 2 tbsp coconut aminos
- 1/4 cup olive oil
- 1/4 tsp fresh grated ginger

Directions

1. In a salad bowl, mix the cabbage with the almonds, vinegar, coconut aminos, oil, and ginger Mix well and serve as a side dish.
2. Enjoy!

Nutrition

Calories: 391, **Fat:** 33.4 g, **Carbs:** 12.7 g, **Protein:** 10 g

28. Healthy Fruit Salad with Yogurt Cream

10 minutes   0 minutes   4

Ingredients

- 1 cup plain Greek yogurt
- 2 tbsp honey
- 1 tsp vanilla extract
- 1 cup diced fresh mango
- 1 cup diced fresh strawberries
- 1 cup diced fresh kiwi

Directions

1. In a medium bowl, whisk together the yogurt, honey, and vanilla extract until combined.
2. In a large bowl, combine the mango, strawberries, and kiwi.
3. Pour the yogurt mixture over the fruit and gently stir to combine.
4. Serve immediately or refrigerate until ready to serve.

Nutrition

Calories: 99, **Protein:** 4.4 g, **Carbs:** 18.7 g, **Fat:** 0.4 g

29. Cabbage and Scallions Salad

10 minutes   0 minutes   4

Ingredients

- 3 scallions, chopped
- 1 green cabbage head, shredded
- 2 carrots, chopped
- 1/2 cup chopped cilantro
- 3 tbsp sunflower seeds
- 2 tbsp sesame seeds
- 1/4 cup balsamic vinegar
- 3 1/2 tbsp olive oil
- 1 tbsp maple syrup

Directions

1. In a salad bowl, mix the cabbage with the scallions, carrots, cilantro, vinegar, oil, maple syrup, sunflower, and sesame seeds. Toss everything together well and serve as a side dish.
2. Enjoy!

Nutrition

Calories: 291, **Fat:** 24.4 g, **Carbs:** 13.6 g, **Protein:** 4.4 g

30. Summertime Fruit Salad

10 minutes   0 minutes   4

Ingredients

- 1 cup diced mango
- 1 cup diced strawberries
- 1 cup diced kiwi
- 1 cup diced cantaloupe
- 2 tbsp honey
- 1/4 tsp ground ginger

Directions

1. In a large bowl, combine the mango, strawberries, kiwi, and cantaloupe.
2. In a small bowl, whisk together the honey, ginger, and turmeric.
3. Serve chilled or at room temperature.

Nutrition

Calories: 75, **Protein:** 1 g, **Carbs:** 16.6 g, **Fat:** 0.4 g

31. Cranberry Salad

15 minutes   0 minutes   4

Ingredients

- 1 cup apples (peeled and chopped)
- 2 (3 oz) packages of raspberry Jell-O
- 1 can whole cranberry sauce (not jellied)
- 1 cup celery (chopped)
- 1/2 cup unsalted nuts

Directions

1. Jell-O should be mixed according to the package guidelines. Add the cranberry sauce, apples, celery, and nuts after the syrup has cooled and thickened. Refrigerate until the mixture is solid.

Nutrition

Calories: 144, **Carbs:** 13.8 g, **Protein:** 3.3 g, **Fat:** 8.6 g

32. Tuna and Vegetable Salad

5 minutes   0 minutes   2

Ingredients

- 2 oz low-sodium tuna in water
- 2 small celery ribs finely diced
- 1 small carrot shredded
- 1 small scallion, white part only, finely chopped
- 2 tbsp light mayonnaise
- 2 tsp fresh parsley or dill

Directions

1. Mix everything in a bowl and serve.

Nutrition

Calories: 174, **Carbs:** 6.6 g, **Protein:** 8.4 g, **Fat:** 12.7 g

33. Chopped Greek Salad

 10 minutes   0 minutes   4

Ingredients

- 1 tbsp red wine vinegar
- 1 tbsp water
- 1 tsp dried oregano
- 1 tbsp extra-virgin olive oil
- 1 medium cucumber, peeled, seeded, and cut into thin half-moons
- 1 can chickpeas drained and rinsed
- 2 oz crumbled regular rindless goat cheese

Directions

1. Whisk the water, vinegar, and oregano in a bowl. Gradually whisk in the oil. Add the cucumber, and chickpeas and toss well. Sprinkle with goat cheese and serve.

Nutrition

Calories: 132, **Carbs:** 10.8 g, **Protein:** 5.7 g, **Fat:** 7.4 g

34. Cucumber Soup

 10 minutes 0 minutes 2

Ingredients

- 2 cups English cucumbers (peeled and diced)
- 1 cup vegetable broth
- 1/8 cup parsley (diced)
- 1/4 tsp salt
- 1/4 cup Greek yogurt (plain)

Directions

1. Combine all ingredients in a blender (except 1/4 cup of sliced cucumbers). Blend until completely smooth. Serve the soup in four bowls, garnished with additional cucumbers. Serve.

Nutrition

Calories: 54, **Carbs:** 5.4 g, **Protein:** 4.5 g, **Fat:** 1.5 g

35. Smoked Turkey Salad

 10 minutes 0 minutes 4

Ingredients

- 2 mangoes, peeled and cubed
- 4 cups salad greens
- 1 cup smoked turkey, sliced
- 1/4 cup cilantro, chopped
- 2 tbsp extra virgin organic olive oil
- 2 tbsp water

Directions

1. In a salad bowl, combine the mangoes with salad greens, turkey, and cilantro and toss.
2. In another bowl, combine the oil using the water and ginger, whisk well, improve the salad, toss, and serve for lunch.
3. Enjoy!

Nutrition

Calories: 207, **Fat:** 8.7 g, **Carbs:** 14.2 g, **Protein:** 17.8 g

36. Pork Salad

10 minutes   35 minutes   6

Ingredients

- 1 lb pork tenderloin, cut into small slices
- 6 sage leaves, chopped
- 1/2 tsp cumin, ground
- 1 tbsp organic essential olive oil
- 1 green lettuce head, torn
- 1 avocado, peeled, pitted, and cubed
- 1 cup canned black beans, no-salt-added, drained and rinsed

For the vinaigrette:
- 1 red sweet pepper, halved
- 1 jalapeno, halved
- 2 tbsp using apple cider vinegar
- 2 tbsp organic olive oil

Directions

1. In a bowl, combine the pork slices with sage, and cumin and toss as well as leave aside for 10 minutes.
2. Heat a pan with 1 tbsp oil over medium-high heat, add pork slices, cook them for 5 minutes on them, and transfer them using a plate.
3. Arrange sweet pepper halves and jalapeno having a lined baking sheet, introduce in the oven, bake at 425°F for 25 minutes, cool them down, peel, and place them in your food processor.
4. Add vinegar and a pair of tbsp oil and pulse well.
5. In a salad bowl, combine the lettuce with avocado, and black beans, toss, and divide between plates.
6. To this mix with pork slices, drizzle the vinaigrette across, and serve for lunch.
7. Enjoy!

Nutrition

Calories: 295, **Fat:** 22.6 g, **Carbs:** 4.1 g, **Protein:** 18.7 g

37. Veggie Lunch Salad

 10 minutes   15 minutes   4

Ingredients

- 1 lb firm tofu, drained and cubed
- 3/4 cup low-fat Italian dressing
- 1 tbsp essential organic olive oil
- 12 oz yellow squash, cubed
- 1/2 cup cooked quinoa
- 1/2 cup sorrel leaves, torn

Directions

1. Heat increase kitchen grill over medium-high heat, add tofu, grill for 5 minutes, and transfer to your salad bowl.
2. Heat a pan with all the oil over medium-high heat, add squash and quinoa, stir, and cook for 10 minutes.
3. Transfer to the bowl with all the tofu, add sorrel leaves and Italian dressing, toss, and serve for lunch.
4. Enjoy!

Nutrition

Calories: 246, **Fat:** 10.6 g, **Carbs:** 20.1 g, **Protein:** 17.4 g

38. Carrot Cucumber Salad

 15 minutes   0 minutes   1

Ingredients

- 1/4 cup rice vinegar, seasoned
- 1/2 tsp olive oil
- 1 tsp stevia
- 1/4 tsp ginger, grated & peeled
- 1/4 tsp salt
- 1 cup carrot, sliced
- 1/2 cucumber, seeded, halved, and sliced

Directions

1. Whisk the stevia, rice vinegar, ginger, salt, and olive oil together in your bowl.
2. Now toss the carrot and cucumber into this mixture.
3. Coat evenly. Plastic wrap the bowl.
4. Keep in the refrigerator for about 30 minutes.

Nutrition

Calories: 175, **Carbs:** 20.9 g, **Fat:** 8.5 g, **Protein:** 3.3 g

39. Cauliflower Soup

10 minutes   50 minutes   4

Ingredients

- 3 lb cauliflower, florets separated
- 1 tbsp coconut oil
- 2 carrots, chopped
- 2 cups beef stock
- 1 cup water
- 1/2 cup coconut milk
- 1 tsp olive oil
- 2 tbsp parsley, chopped

Directions

1. Heat a pot with all the coconut oil over medium-high heat, and add carrots. Stir and cook for 5 minutes.
2. Add cauliflower, water, and stock, stir, bring to a boil, cover, and cook for 45 minutes.
3. Transfer soup to your blender and pulse well, add coconut milk, pulse well again, ladle into bowls, drizzle the essential olive oil on the soup, sprinkle parsley, and serve for lunch.
4. Enjoy!

Nutrition

Calories: 253, **Fat:** 14.8 g, **Carbs:** 15.5 g, **Protein:** 14.3 g

40. Purple Potato Soup

10 minutes   1 hour 15   6

minutes

Ingredients

- 6 purple potatoes, chopped
- 1 cauliflower head, florets separated
- 3 tbsp extra virgin olive oil
- 1 tbsp thyme, chopped
- 1 leek, chopped
- 2 shallots, chopped
- 4 cups chicken stock, low-sodium

Directions

1. In a baking dish, mix potatoes with cauliflower, thyme, and half of the oil, toss to coat, introduce inside the oven, and bake for 45 minutes at 400°F.
2. Heat a pot while using the remaining oil over medium-high heat, add leeks and shallots, stir, and cook for ten mins.
3. Add roasted veggies and stock, stir, give a boil, cook for twenty minutes, transfer soup to your meal processor, blend well, divide into bowls, and serve.
4. Enjoy!

Nutrition

Calories: 183, **Fat:** 8.9 g, **Carbs:** 20.9 g, **Protein:** 5.5 g

41. Broccoli Soup

 10 minutes 1 hour 4

Ingredients

- 2 lb broccoli, florets separated
- 1 tbsp essential olive oil
- 1 cup celery, chopped
- 2 carrots, chopped
- 3 and 1/2 cups of low-sodium chicken stock
- 1 tbsp chopped cilantro

Directions

1. Heat a pot with all the oil over medium-high heat, add the celery, carrots, and chicken stock stir, and cook for 5 minutes.
2. Add broccoli stir and cook over medium heat for 1 hour.
3. Pulse using an immersion blender, add cilantro, stir the soup again, divide into bowls, and serve.
4. Enjoy!

Nutrition

Calories: 131, **Fat:** 5 g, **Carbs:** 12.1 g, **Protein:** 9.6 g

42. Leeks Soup

 10 minutes 30 minutes 4

Ingredients

- 2 gold potatoes, chopped
- 1 cup cauliflower florets
- 5 leeks, chopped
- 3 tbsp essential organic olive oil
- Handful parsley chopped
- 4 cups low-sodium chicken stock

Directions

1. Heat a pot with all the oil over medium-high heat.
2. Add potatoes, cauliflower, leeks, and stock, stir, bring to some simmer, cook over medium heat for thirty minutes, blend with an immersion blender, add parsley, stir, ladle into bowls, and serve.
3. Enjoy!

Nutrition

Calories: 230, **Fat:** 12.6 g, **Carbs:** 21.3 g, **Protein:** 8 g

43. Mesmerizing Lentil Soup

 10 minutes 8 hours 8

Ingredients

- 1 lb dried lentils, soaked overnight and rinsed
- 3 carrots, peeled and chopped
- 1 celery stalk, chopped
- 6 cups vegetable broth
- 1 tsp ground cumin
- 1/4 tsp salt
- 1 tsp dried thyme
- 1/4 tsp liquid smoke

Directions

1. Add the listed ingredients to Slow Cooker and stir well. Place lid and cook for 8 hours on low heat. Stir and serve

Nutrition

Calories: 449, **Fat:** 3.8 g, **Carbs:** 71.6 g, **Protein:** 32.4 g

44. Cream of Mushroom Soup

10 minutes   10 minutes   5

Ingredients

- 1 1/2 cups fresh mushrooms, sliced
- 2 tbsp unsalted butter
- 2 cans chicken broth, less/ reduced sodium
- 6 tbsp all-purpose flour
- 1 cup half-and-half cream, fat-free
- A pinch of salt

Directions

1. Heat butter in a large saucepan and overheat. Sauté mushrooms until tender. Add the ingredients, including flour, salt, and one can of broth, and mix them well until it becomes smooth. Stir in the mushroom mixture. Stir in the remaining broth. Boil and cook until thickened for about 2 minutes. Reduce the heat and stir in the cream. Simmer, uncovered, until flavors are blended, about 10 minutes. Serve and enjoy.

Nutrition

Calories: 219, **Carbs:** 10.8 g, **Protein:** 4.6 g, **Fat:** 17.5 g

45. Roasted Vegetable Soup

 15 minutes 20 minutes 4

Ingredients

- 1 tbsp olive oil
- 2 lb Potatoes diced (1 cm thick)
- 2 yellow bell peppers, diced
- 1/2 tsp fresh rosemary, finely chopped
- 1 carrot, halved lengthwise and cut into 1 cm piece
- 2/5 quarts of carrot juice
- 1 tsp fresh tarragon
- 1 tsp salt

Directions

1. Preheat the oven to 400°F. Place the carrot, potatoes, and bell peppers in a baking tray. Drizzle with olive oil and roast for 10 to 15 minutes. In a saucepan, add carrot juice and tarragon; let boil a little. Add all roasted vegetables and stir well. Let it simmer for a few minutes. Season with salt and rosemary. Mix well. Serve and enjoy.

Nutrition

Calories: 278, **Carbs:** 49.2 g, **Protein:** 6.1 g, **Fat:** 6.3 g

46. Quick Spinach Salad

 10 minutes 0 minutes 2

Ingredients

- 1/2 lb baby spinach
- 1 Hass avocado, peeled, pitted, and sliced
- 3 tbsp Pistou

Directions

1. In a medium-sized bowl, Place all of the ingredients together.
2. Serve right away.

Nutrition

Calories: 303, **Fat:** 27.2 g, **Protein:** 8.9 g, **Carbs:** 5.4 g

47. Root Vegetable Salad with Maple Syrup Dressing

25 minutes　　0 minutes　　4

Ingredients

For the dressing:
- 1/4 cup olive oil
- 1 tsp grated fresh ginger
- 2 tbsp apple cider vinegar
- 3 tbsp pure maple syrup
- 1 tsp Sea salt

For the slaw:
- 5 radishes, shredded
- 2 carrots, shredded, or 1 cup shredded packaged carrots
- 1 jicama, or 2 parsnips, peeled and shredded
- 1/2 celeriac peeled and shredded
- 1/4 fennel bulb, shredded
- 2 scallions, white and green parts, peeled and thinly sliced
- 1/2 cup pumpkin seeds, roasted

Directions

To make the dressing:
1. Add the dressing ingredients, except the sea salt, into a small bowl, and whisk them together until well blended. With sea salt to season, set it aside.

To make the slaw:
1. Add the slaw ingredients, except the pumpkin seeds into a large bowl, and toss them together.
2. Pour in the dressing and coat well.
3. Place the pumpkin seeds over the slaw, and serve.

Nutrition

Calories: 214, **Fat:** 14 g, **Protein:** 2 g, **Carbs:** 20 g

48. Mackerel Soup

10 minutes   40 minutes   4

Ingredients

- 4 mackerel fillets, skinless, boneless and cubed
- 2 lemongrass sticks, chopped
- 1 tbsp coconut oil
- 12 oz coconut milk
- 4 cups vegetable stock
- A handful of coriander, chopped

Directions

1. Heat a pot with the coconut oil over medium-high heat, add lemongrass, stir, and cook for 3 minutes. Add coconut milk, stock, and mackerel, stir, and bring to a boil. Reduce heat to low and simmer for 35 minutes. Add coriander, stir, and let the soup sit for 10 minutes. Ladle it into bowls and serve.
2. Enjoy!

Nutrition

Calories: 396, **Fat:** 33.8 g, **Carbs:** 3.6 g, **Protein:** 19.6 g

49. Kale Soup

10 minutes   20 minutes   4

Ingredients

- 1 tsp olive oil
- 3 sweet potatoes, chopped
- 4 cups chicken stock
- 1 lb kale, chopped
- A pinch of sea salt

Directions

1. Heat a pot with the oil over medium heat. Add stock and sweet potatoes, stir, bring to a simmer, and cook for 15 minutes. Blend using an immersion blender, add kale, and salt, cook everything for 4 minutes more, ladle into bowls, and serve.
2. Enjoy!

Nutrition

Calories: 202, **Fat:** 5.8 g, **Carbs:** 29.8 g, **Protein:** 7.7 g

50. Eggplant Salad

10 minutes   30 minutes   3

Ingredients

- 2 eggplants (peeled and sliced)
- 1/2 cup egg-free mayonnaise
- 2 green bell pepper (sliced and remove seeds)
- 1/2 cup fresh parsley
- 1 tsp salt

Directions

1. Preheat the oven to 480°F. After that, put the eggplants and bell pepper in a baking pan. Bake the veggies for approximately 30 minutes, flipping halfway through. Then, combine the cooked veggies with the other ingredients in a mixing dish. Mix thoroughly. Serve.

Nutrition

Calories: 275, **Carbs:** 10.8 g, **Protein:** 4.3 g, **Fat:** 23.9 g

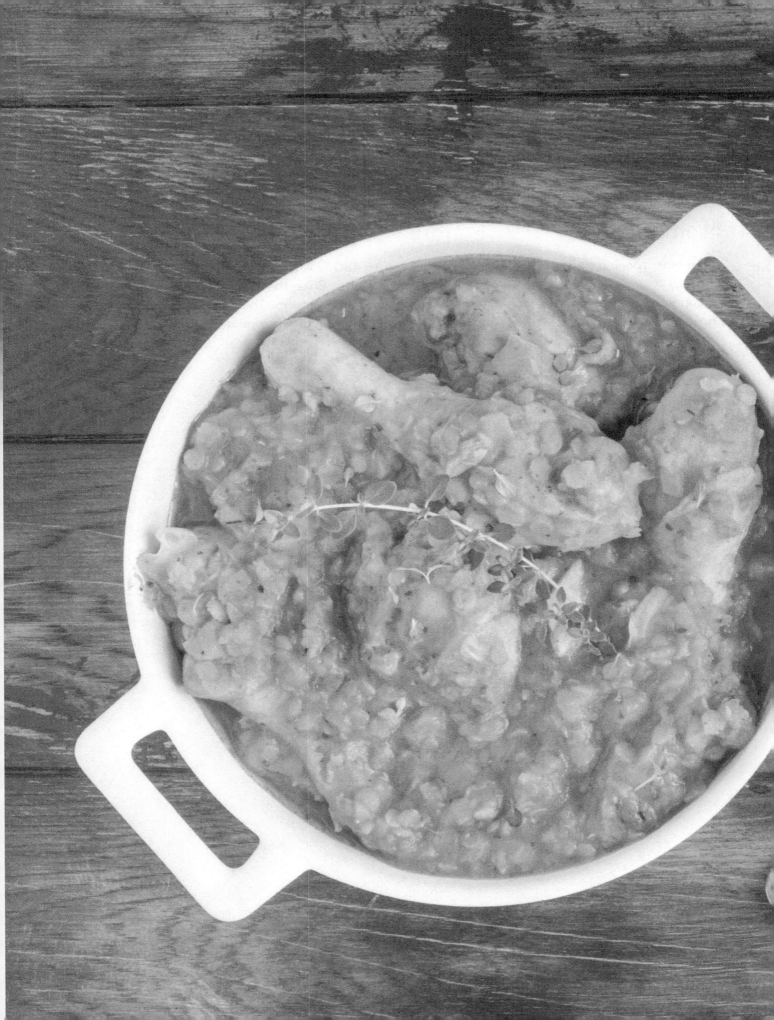

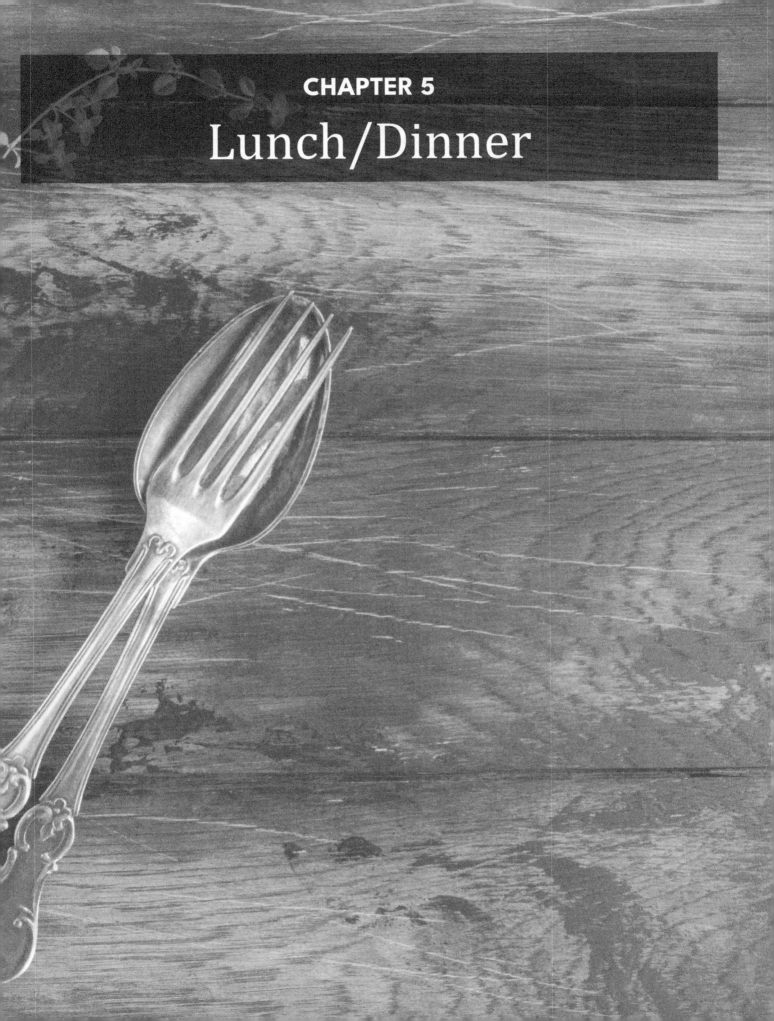

CHAPTER 5
Lunch/Dinner

51. Chicken with Parsley Sauce

30 minutes   40 minutes   6

Ingredients

- 1 cup chopped parsley
- 1 tsp dried oregano
- 1/2 cup olive oil
- 1/4 cup vegetable stock
- A pinch of salt
- 12 chicken thighs

Directions

1. In your food processor, mix parsley with oregano, salt, oil, and the stock. Pulse well until smooth. In a bowl, mix the chicken with the parsley sauce and toss, cover, and keep in the fridge for 30 minutes. Heat your kitchen grill over medium heat and place the chicken pieces on the grill. Close the lid and cook for 20 minutes. Flip the chicken and cook for 20 minutes more. Divide between plates and serve with the parsley sauce on top.
2. Enjoy!

Nutrition

Calories: 541, **Fat:** 44.7 g, **Carbs:** 0 g, **Protein:** 34.8 g

52. Chicken and Lentil Casserole

10 minutes   1 hour and   8

40 minutes

Ingredients

- 1 1/2 cups green lentils
- 3 cups clean chicken stock
- 2 lb chicken breasts, skinless, boneless and cubed
- A pinch of Sea salt
- 3 tsp ground cumin
- Cooking spray
- 2 carrots, chopped
- 2 cups corn
- 1 cup chopped parsley

Directions

1. Put the stock in a pot, and add a pinch of salt and the lentils. Stir, bring to a boil over medium heat, cover, and simmer for 35 minutes.
2. Heat a pan with some cooking spray over medium-high heat and add the chicken, season with salt, and 1 tsp cumin.
3. Cook for 5 minutes on each side then transfer to a bowl.
4. Heat the pan again over medium heat, add carrots, salt, and 1 tsp cumin. Stir, cook for 7 minutes, and transfer to the bowl with the chicken.
5. Drain the lentils, and add them to the bowl with the meat and then the rest of the cumin, corn, and parsley.
6. Toss, transfer the whole mix to a baking dish and place in the oven at 350°F, and bake for 50 minutes. Divide between plates and serve.
7. Enjoy!

Nutrition
Calories: 280, **Fat:** 2.9 g, **Carbs:** 33.4 g, **Protein:** 30.1 g

53. Herb Lamb

10 minutes   20 minutes   6

Ingredients

- 14 oz Lamb neck fillet, trimmed of sinew and excess fat
- 1/2 tbsp cumin
- 1/2 tbsp ground coriander
- 1 tbsp toasted coriander seed, bashed
- 2 tbsp olive oil, plus a drizzle
- 1 bunch of dill, chopped
- 1 bunch of coriander leaves picked
- 2 cups feta
- 1 pomegranate, seeds only

Directions

1. Set the oven to 400°F.
2. Season the lamb with spices.
3. Heat oil in a suitable frying pan and sear the lamb for 3 minutes per side.
4. Place it on a baking sheet and roast for 10 minutes in the oven.
5. Top the lamb with the remaining ingredients and serve.

Nutrition

Calories: 338, **Fat:** 25.2 g, **Carbs:** 7.3 g, **Protein:** 20.6 g

54. Split Pea Soup with Coconut

 25 minutes   1 hour 10   8

minutes

Ingredients

Soup:

- 2 tbsp oil
- 4 chopped carrots
- 1 tsp Kosher salt
- 1 tsp fennel seeds
- 2 tsp curry powder Madras
- 1 tsp mustard seeds
- 12 oz split peas (yellow)

Coconut and assembly:

- 1/2 tsp coriander seeds
- 1/2 tsp fennel seeds
- 1/2 tsp mustard seeds
- 2 tsp oil olive, vegetable, or coconut
- 1/4 cup coconut flakes unsweetened

Directions

The soup:

1. Heat the oil in a large, heavy saucepan set over medium heat. Add the carrots, sprinkle with a bit of salt, and simmer, often stirring, for approximately 5 minutes or until the veggies are very mushy and only have a slight color at the ends. Use a pestle and mortar to lightly crush or finely chop the fennel seeds. Curry, fennel seeds, and mustard seeds are cooked in a skillet with steady stirring for less than one minute until fragrant (mustard seeds will begin to explode).
2. In a mixing bowl, add the separated peas, toss to coat, and then add enough water and stock to make four cups. For 50 to 55 minutes, or when the split peas are very mushy, and other peas are beginning to split, increase the heat to a low simmer, then bring to a boil, stirring regularly and adding additional water if the soup seems too thick.
3. Use a potato masher to mash the soup until the split peas are tiny and the consistency is textured yet creamy (using an immersion for a smoother soup directly blend in the pot). If required, add more salt to the dish.

Assembly coconut:

1. Lightly crush the fennel, mustard seeds, and cilantro while the soup is heating.
2. Heat the oil in a low-temperature pan. Cook the spices and coconut flakes while stirring regularly for about a minute or until the coconut becomes golden brown and the spices start to crackle. Place on a dish, sprinkle with salt, and let to cool (as it cools, the coconut will be crisp).
3. On top of the soup, garnish with coriander and spiced coconut.

Nutrition
Calories: 170, **Fat:** 12.4 g, **Carbs:** 10.4 g, **Protein:** 4.3 g

55. Balsamic Scallops

5 minutes   10 or so   4

minutes

Ingredients

- 1 lb sea scallops
- 4 scallions, chopped
- 2 tbsp olive oil
- 1 tbsp balsamic vinegar
- 1 tbsp cilantro, chopped
- A pinch of salt

Directions

1. Heat a pan with the oil over medium-high heat, and add the scallops, the scallions, and the other ingredients.
2. Toss, cook for 10 minutes, divide into bowls, and serve.

Nutrition

Calories: 233, **Fat:** 9.1 g, **Carbs:** 10.2 g, **Protein:** 27.9 g

56. Coconut Zucchini Cream

10 minutes   25 minutes   4

Ingredients

- 3 zucchinis, cut into medium chunks
- 2 tbsp coconut milk
- 4 cups chicken stock
- 2 tbsp olive oil
- A pinch of sea salt

Directions

1. Heat a pot with the oil over medium heat. Add zucchini, stir, and cook for 5 minutes. Add stock and salt, then stir. Bring to a boil, cover the pot, and simmer the soup for 20 minutes. Mix with the coconut milk, blend using an immersion blender, ladle into bowls, and serve.
2. Enjoy!

Nutrition

Calories: 112, **Fat:** 9.6 g, **Carbs:** 2.3 g, **Protein:** 4.3 g

57. Tender Coconut Chicken

15 minutes   35 minutes   4

Ingredients

- 2 tbsp ginger, grated
- 1 tbsp raw honey
- 1 1/2 cups unsweetened coconut milk
- 1/2 tsp ground cardamom
- 1 tbsp olive oil
- 1 lb chicken thighs, bone-in, skin-on
- 1 scallion, chopped

Directions

1. In a bowl, whisk the ginger, honey, coconut milk, and cardamom, and set aside.
2. Place a large skillet over medium-high heat, and pour the olive oil.
3. Add chicken thighs to pan sear, and cook for about 20 minutes, until golden.
4. Pour a bowl with the coconut milk, ginger, and honey over the chicken, and bring the liquid to a boil. Reduce the heat to simmer, and cover for about 15 minutes until cooked through.
5. Garnished with scallions.
6. Enjoy.

Nutrition

Calories: 418, **Fat:** 23.9 g, **Protein:** 46.7 g, **Carbs:** 4 g

58. Vegetarian Pizza with Autumn Toppings

15 minutes   15 minutes   4

Ingredients

For the crust:
- 2/3 cup whole wheat flour
- 1/2 tbsp dried yeast
- 2 tsp brown sugar
- 1 tbsp extra virgin olive oil
- 2/3 cup warm water
- 1/2 tsp salt
- 1 tbsp cornmeal

For the toppings:
- 1 cup roasted pumpkin cubes
- 2 tsp passata
- 5 Lacinato kale leaves chopped
- 1/4 cup lightly toasted walnuts
- 1 tsp honey
- 2 tsp extra virgin olive oil
- 1/2 pomegranate seeds

Directions

1. Water, sugar, and yeast are mixed in a bowl; the yeast should dissolve after 10 minutes.
2. In a large mixing basin, combine the salt and flour, add the yeast mixture, drizzle in the olive oil, and whisk with a fork.
3. When an elastic dough develops, transfer the ingredients to a floured surface and knead for approximately 5 minutes. Add 1 more tbsp of flour if the mixture is too wet.
4. The dough should be placed on a dish, covered with a cloth, and let to rise for 30 minutes at room temperature.
5. Turn the oven's temperature up to 200°F.
6. Pizza dough should be shaped into an oval or narrow circular.
7. Place the cornmeal over the pizza dough on a cookie sheet covered with bakery release paper.
8. Spread the passata thinly on top of the pizza crust before adding the minced kale and pumpkin.
9. After baking for 15 minutes, remove from oven and top with pomegranate seeds and walnuts.
10. Serve heated after adding honey.

Nutrition
Calories: 288, **Fat:** 15.8 g, **Carbs:** 31.1 g, **Protein:** 5.2 g

59. Tender Stir-Fry Chicken

 15 minutes   15 minutes   2

Ingredients

- 3 tbsp extra-virgin olive oil
- 1 lb boneless, skinless chicken breasts, cut into bite-size pieces
- 1 cup broccoli florets
- 6 scallions, white and green parts, chopped
- 1 recipe stir-fry sauce
- 2 tbsp sesame seeds toasted

Directions

1. In a nonstick skillet, warm over medium-high heat to heat the olive oil, until it shimmers.
2. Combine the chicken, broccoli, and scallions, cook for 5 to 7 minutes, and stir until cooked through.
3. Arrange the stir-fry sauce, cook for 5 minutes, and stir until the sauce reduces.
4. Garnish with sesame seeds.
5. Enjoy.

Nutrition

Calories: 324, **Fat:** 30.4 g, **Protein:** 6.3 g, **Carbs:** 7.1 g

60. Tuna Stew

 10 minutes   35 minutes   4

Ingredients

- 1 tbsp olive oil
- 1/4 pint chicken stock
- 3 sweet potatoes, cubed
- 2 tuna fillets, flaked
- 1 tbsp chopped coriander

Directions

1. Heat a pot with the oil over medium heat. Add the stock, potatoes, and paprika. Stir, bring to a simmer, and cook for 20 minutes over medium heat. Add the tuna, cook for 10 minutes more, divide into bowls, sprinkle coriander on top, and serve.
2. Enjoy!

Nutrition

Calories: 184, **Fat:** 8 g, **Carbs:** 16 g, **Protein:** 11.8 g

61. Thyme Chard-Turkey Burgers

10 minutes   12 minutes   4

Ingredients

- 2 cups fresh chard, washed
- 1 lb ground turkey
- 1/2 tsp green pepper flakes
- 1/2 tsp salt
- 1/2 tsp dried dill
- 1/4 tsp dried thyme
- 1 tbsp olive oil

Directions

1. Process the chard for about 15 seconds until the vegetables are minced.
2. Add the turkey, dill, thyme, pepper flakes, and salt. Process for 20 to 30 seconds until well mixed.
3. Form the turkey mixture into four patties.
4. Coat a large skillet over medium heat with the olive oil. Add the patties and cook each side for about 6 minutes.

Nutrition

Calories: 209, **Fat:** 11.4 g, **Protein:** 21 g, **Carbs:** 5.9 g

62. Easy Turkey Meatloaf

5 minutes   25 minutes   6

Ingredients

- 18 oz ground turkey breast
- 3 carrots, peeled and grated
- 1 egg beaten
- 1 tbsp soy sauce
- 1 tbsp Dijon mustard
- 1 tsp fish sauce
- 1 tsp dried thyme
- 1 tsp dried rosemary

Directions

1. Preheat the oven to 350˚F.
2. Mix the turkey, carrots, egg soy sauce, mustard, fish sauce, thyme, and rosemary in a large bowl. Evenly divide the meat-loaf mixture among the cups of a nonstick 6-muffin tin.
3. Bake for about 25 minutes until cooked through.

Nutrition

Calories: 149, **Fat:** 6.3 g, **Carbs:** 6.5 g, **Protein:** 16.6 g

63. Rosemary Broiled Shrimp

10 minutes   4 minutes   6

Ingredients

- 3/4 lb large shrimps, shelled and deveined
- 1 tsp Extra virgin olive oil
- 1 tsp Himalayan crystal salt, to taste
- 1/2 tsp dried rosemary, crushed

Directions

1. Preheat the broiler and place the rack 4 inches from the heat. Line a baking tray with foil.
2. Place the shrimp on the prepared baking tray in a single layer. Drizzle with the oil. With the rosemary and salt, sprinkle over the shrimp.
3. Broil for about 3 to 4 minutes. Remove from the heat and serve.

Nutrition

Calories: 238, **Fat:** 4.4 g, **Carbs:** 8.9 g, **Protein:** 40.8 g

64. Chicken and Pumpkin Stew

10 minutes   8 hours   4

Ingredients

- 2 carrots, chopped
- 2 celery sticks, chopped
- 2 sweet potatoes, cubed
- 30 oz canned pumpkin puree
- 2 quarts chicken stock
- 2 cups chicken meat, skinless, boneless, and shredded
- A pinch of sea salt
- 1/4 cup ground arrowroot

Directions

1. In your slow cooker, mix carrots, celery, sweet potatoes, pumpkin puree, chicken, stock, salt, and ground arrowroot. Stir, cover, and cook on Low for 8 hours. Uncover the slow cooker, stir, divide the stew into bowls, and serve.
2. Enjoy!

Nutrition

Calories: 191, **Fat:** 3 g, **Carbs:** 23.2 g, **Protein:** 17.9 g

65. Turkey Stew

15 minutes   22 minutes   2

Ingredients

- 1 tsp extra virgin olive oil
- 1 celery stalk, minced
- 1/4 tsp Freshly ground coriander
- 1/2 tsp freshly ground cumin
- 1/2 lb lean ground turkey
- 1/2 cup Low-sodium Vegetable Broth
- 1 tsp Himalayan crystal salt, to taste

Directions

1. In a pan, heat the oil on medium heat. Add the celery and sauté for 4 minutes. Add the coriander and cumin, and sauté for a further minute.
2. Add the turkey and cook, stirring, for 6 to 7 minutes. Add the remaining ingredients. Increase the heat and bring the pan to a boil. Once boiling, cover and simmer for about 8 to 10 minutes.

Nutrition

Calories: 232, **Fat:** 15 g, **Carbs:** 3.6 g, **Protein:** 20.7 g

66. Pork Chops and Sauce

10 minutes   9 hours   6

Ingredients

- 6 pork loin chops
- 1 tbsp extra-virgin organic olive oil
- 2 tbsp tapioca, crushed
- 10 oz low-sodium cream of mushroom soup
- 1/2 cup apple juice
- 2 tsp thyme, chopped
- 1 1/2 cups mushrooms, sliced

Directions

1. Heat a pan when using oil over medium-high heat, add pork chops, brown them for 4 minutes, and transfer to a slow cooker.
2. Add crushed tapioca, cream of mushroom soup, apple juice, thyme, and mushrooms, toss, cover, and cook on Low for 9 hours.
3. Divide the pork chops and sauce between plates and serve.
4. Enjoy!

Nutrition

Calories: 372, **Fat:** 18.8 g, **Carbs:** 6.4 g, **Protein:** 44.5 g

67. Seafood Noodles

10 minutes   20 minutes   4

Ingredients

- 8 oz whole wheat noodles
- 2 tbsp olive oil
- 1/2 tsp ground ginger
- 1/2 tsp ground turmeric
- 1/4 tsp sea salt
- 1/2 cup of vegetable broth
- 1/2 cup of coconut milk
- 1/2 lb shrimp, peeled and deveined
- 1/2 lb scallops
- 1/2 cup frozen peas

Directions

1. Cook the noodles according to the package instructions. Drain and set aside.
2. Heat the olive oil in a large skillet over medium heat.
3. Add the ginger, turmeric, and sea salt and cook for 1 minute, stirring constantly.
4. Add the vegetable broth, coconut milk, shrimp, and scallops, and cook for 5 minutes, stirring occasionally.
5. Add the cooked noodles and frozen peas and cook for an additional 2 minutes, stirring occasionally.

Nutrition

Calories: 411, **Protein:** 23.8 g, **Carbs:** 43.9 g, **Fat:** 15.6 g

68. Duck with Bok Choy

 10 minutes 48 minutes 8

Ingredients

- 4 duck legs
- 2 tbsp olive oil
- 2 tbsp fresh ginger, grated
- 2 tbsp tamari sauce
- 2 tbsp honey
- 2 tbsp sesame oil
- 2 bunches of bok choy, chopped
- 2 tbsp sesame seeds
- 1 tsp salt

Directions

1. Preheat the oven to 375°F.
2. Place the duck legs in a baking dish and season with salt. Bake for 30 minutes.
3. Heat the olive oil in a large skillet over medium heat. Add the ginger and cook for 1 minute.
4. Add the tamari sauce, honey, and sesame oil and stir to combine.
5. Add the bok choy and cook for 5 minutes, stirring occasionally.
6. Add the sesame seeds and cook for an additional 2 minutes.
7. Remove the duck legs from the oven and top them with the bok choy mixture. Bake for an additional 10 minutes.
8. Serve the duck legs with the bok choy.

Nutrition

Calories: 310, **Protein:** 28.6 g, **Carbs:** 4.9 g, **Fat:** 19.6 g

69. Deliciously Simple Beef

 10 minutes   10 hours   4

Ingredients

- 1 large onion, sliced thinly
- 1/4 cup extra-virgin olive oil
- 1 tsp oregano, dried
- Salt and black pepper, freshly ground, to taste
- 2 lb beef chuck roast, cut into bite-sized pieces

Directions

1. In a slow cooker, place all the ingredients except for beef cubes and stir to combine.
2. Add the beef cubes and stir to combine.
3. Set the slow cooker on "Low" and cook, covered for about 8–10 hours.
4. Serve hot.

Nutrition

Calories: 377, **Carbs:** 1.9 g, **Protein:** 48.3 g, **Fat:** 19.5 g

70. Holiday Feast Lamb Shanks

15 minutes   8 hours 5

8

minutes

Ingredients

- 4 lamb shanks
- Salt and black pepper, freshly ground, to taste
- 1 tbsp olive oil
- 1 lb baby potatoes, halved
- 1 cup Kalamata olives
- 1 cup chicken broth
- 2 1/2 tsp oregano, dried
- 1 tsp rosemary, dried
- 1 tsp basil, dried
- 1 tsp onion powder

Directions

1. Season the lamb shanks with salt and black pepper evenly.
2. In a large heavy-bottomed skillet, heat the olive oil over medium-high heat and sear the lamb shanks for about 4–5 minutes or until browned completely.
3. Remove from the heat.
4. In a slow cooker, place the potatoes, olives, salt, and broth place the lamb on top and sprinkle with dried herbs and onion powder.
5. Set the slow cooker on "Low" and cook, covered for about 8 hours.
6. Serve hot.

Nutrition

Calories: 467, **Carbs:** 20.8 g, **Protein:** 31.5 g, **Fat:** 28.8 g

71. Beef Steaks with Creamy Bacon and Mushrooms

10 minutes   40 minutes   4

Ingredients

- 2 oz bacon, chopped
- 1 cup mushrooms, sliced
- 1 shallot, chopped
- 1 cup heavy cream
- 1 lb beef steaks
- 1 tsp ground nutmeg
- 1/4 cup coconut oil
- Salt and black pepper to taste
- 1 tbsp parsley chopped

Directions

1. Set a frying pan at medium heat, then cook the bacon for 2 to 3 minutes and set aside. In the same pan, warm the oil, add in the onions, and mushrooms, and cook for 4 minutes. Stir in the beef, season with salt, black pepper, and nutmeg, and sear until browned, about 2 minutes per side.
2. Preheat oven to 360°F and insert the pan in the oven to bake for 25 minutes. Remove the beefsteaks to a bowl and cover with foil.
3. Place the pan over medium heat, pour in the heavy cream over the mushroom mixture, add in the reserved bacon, and cook for 5 minutes; remove from heat. Spread the bacon/mushroom sauce over beefsteaks, sprinkle with parsley, and serve.

Nutrition

Calories: 471, **Fat:** 38.7 g, **Carbs:** 3.6 g, **Protein:** 27.2 g

72. Cilantro Beef Curry with Cauliflower

 6 minutes 15 minutes 3

Ingredients

- 1 tbsp olive oil
- 1/2 lb ground beef
- 1 tsp turmeric
- 1 tbsp cilantro, chopped
- 1 tbsp ginger paste
- 1/2 tsp garam masala
- 1 head cauliflower, cut into florets
- Salt and chili pepper to taste
- 1/4 cup water

Directions

1. Warm oil in a saucepan at medium heat, and put the beef, ginger paste, and garam masala in. Cook for 5 minutes while breaking any lumps.
2. Stir in the cauliflower, season with salt, turmeric, and chili pepper, and cook covered for 6 minutes. Add the water and bring to a boil over medium heat for 10 minutes or until the water has reduced by half. Scoop the curry into serving bowls and serve sprinkled with cilantro.

Nutrition

Calories: 172, **Fat:** 9.2 g, **Carbs:** 3.6 g, **Protein:** 18.9 g

73. Cranberry Pork BBQ Dish

10 minutes   50 minutes   4

Ingredients

- 3–4 lb pork shoulder, boneless, fat trimmed

For sauce:
- 3 tbsp liquid smoke
- 2 cups fresh cranberries
- 1/4 cup hot sauce
- 1/3 cup blackstrap molasses
- 1/2 cup of water
- 1/2 cup apple cider vinegar
- 1 tsp salt
- 1 tbsp adobo sauce
- 1 chipotle pepper in adobo sauce, diced

Directions

1. Cut pork against halves/thirds and keep it on the side
2. Set your Ninja Foodi to sauté mode and let it heat up. Add cranberries and water to the pot
3. Let them simmer for 4 to 5 minutes until cranberries start to pop, add the rest of the sauce ingredients and simmer for 5 minutes more. Add pork to the pot and lock the lid
4. Cook on high pressure for 40 minutes. Quick-release pressure
5. Use a fork to shred the pork and serve it on your favorite greens

Nutrition

Calories: 375, **Fat:** 15.3 g, **Carbs:** 15.6 g, **Protein:** 43.7 g

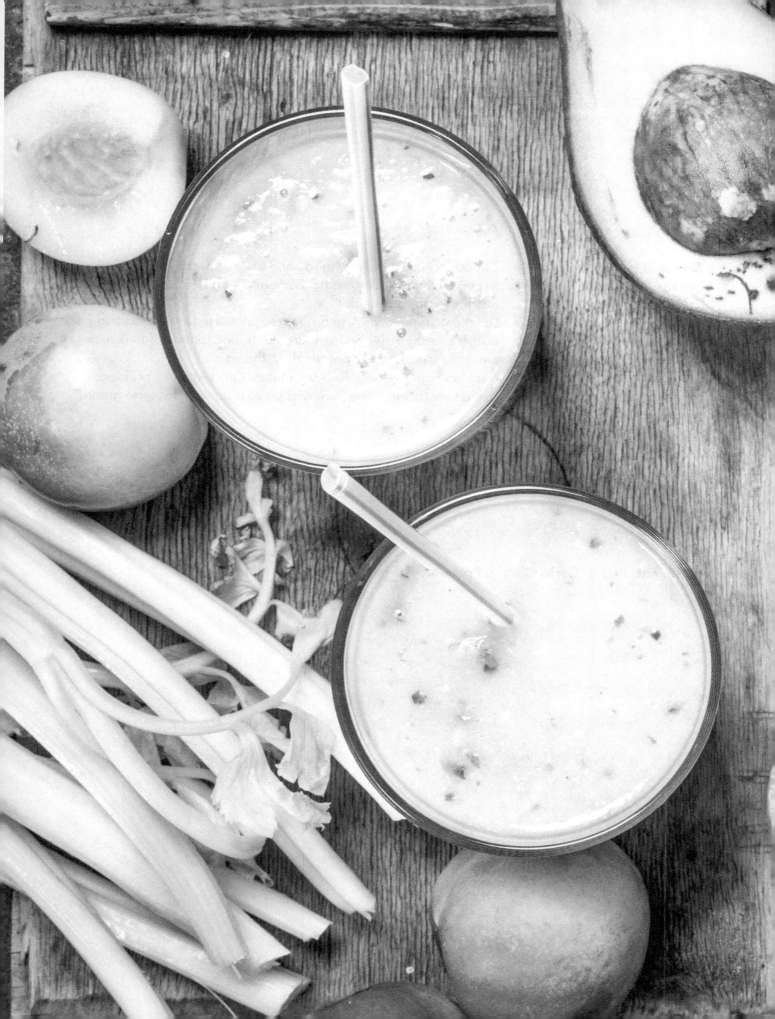

CHAPTER 6

Smoothies

74. Green Smoothie

 10 minutes 0 minutes 4

Ingredients

- 1 cup alkaline water
- 3/4 cup raw coconut water
- 1/2 tsp probiotic powder
- 2 cups firmly packed baby spinach
- 1 cup raw young Thai coconut meat
- 1 avocado, peeled and pitted
- 1/2 cucumber chopped
- 1 tsp Stevia, to taste
- A pinch Celtic sea salt
- 2 cups ice cubes

Directions

1. Add all the ingredients to a blender.
2. Blend well until smooth.
3. Serve with an avocado slice on top.

Nutrition

Calories: 279, **Fat:** 27.2 g, **Carbs:** 4 g, **Protein:** 4.6 g

75. Avocado Smoothie

 10 minutes   0 minutes   3

Ingredients

- 1 carrot, grated
- 1 avocado, cored and peeled
- 1/2 pear, cored
- 1/2 cup blackberries
- 1 1/2 cups unsweetened almond milk

Directions

1. Add all the ingredients to a blender.
2. Blend well until smooth.
3. Serve with blackberries on top.

Nutrition

Calories: 219, **Fat:** 18.3 g, **Carbs:** 9.2 g, **Protein:** 4.4 g

76. Sunshine Smoothie

 5 minutes   0 minutes   1

Ingredients

- 2 1/2 cups frozen strawberries
- 2 cups spinach
- 1 1/4 cups coconut milk
- 1 cup crushed ice

Directions

1. Pour all the ingredients into a food processor. Pulse to purée until creamy and smooth.
2. Serve immediately.

Nutrition

Calories: 227, **Fat:** 14.4 g, **Protein:** 5.9 g, **Carbs:** 18.3 g

77. Pear and Green Tea Smoothie

5 minutes   0 minutes   2

Ingredients

- 2 pears, peeled, cored, and chopped
- 2 cups strongly brewed green tea
- 1 (1-inch) piece fresh ginger, peeled and roughly chopped, or 1 tsp ground ginger
- 2 tbsp raw honey
- 1 cup unsweetened almond milk
- 1 cup crushed ice

Directions

1. Pour all the ingredients into a food processor. Pulse to purée until creamy and smooth.
2. Serve immediately.

Nutrition

Calories: 150, **Fat:** 2.3 g, **Protein:** 1.5 g, **Carbs:** 30 g

78. Refreshing Apple Smoothie

 5 minutes 5 minutes 1

Ingredients

- 1 medium apple, chopped
- 1/4 tsp ground ginger
- 1 scoop vanilla protein powder
- 3/4 cup spinach
- 1 1/2 cups unsweetened almond milk

Directions

1. Add chopped apple and remaining ingredients into the blender and blend until smooth and creamy.

Nutrition

Calories: 289, **Fat:** 2.7 g, **Carbs:** 38.2 g, **Protein:** 24 g

79. Delicious Mango Smoothie

5 minutes   0 minutes   2

Ingredients

- 1 cup mango chunks
- 1/4 tsp turmeric
- 1 tsp vanilla
- 1 banana
- 1 scoop vanilla protein powder
- 1 cup unsweetened almond milk

Directions

1. Add mango chunks and remaining ingredients into the blender and blend until smooth and creamy.
2. Serve immediately and enjoy.

Nutrition

Calories: 216, **Fat:** 2 g, **Carbs:** 29.5 g, **Protein:** 25.4 g

80. Raspberry and Chard Smoothie

5 minutes   0 minute   2

Ingredients

- 2 cups coconut water
- 2 cups Swiss chards
- 2 cups fresh whole raspberries

Directions

1. Whizz all the ingredients on high. Pour into a cup and enjoy.

Nutrition

Calories: 152, **Carbs:** 26.3 g, **Fat:** 7.1 g, **Protein:** 5.4 g

81. Apple and Kale Smoothie

 5 minutes   0 minute   1

Ingredients

- 1 cup spring water
- 2 cups kale leaves, fresh
- 1 large apple, cored

Directions

1. Whizz all the ingredients on high.
2. Pour into a cup and enjoy.

Nutrition

Calories: 121, **Carbs:** 23.1 g, **Fat:** 0.7 g, **Protein:** 5.7 g

82. Banana Alkaline Smoothie

 10 minutes   0 minutes   2

Ingredients

- 1/2 cup coconut water
- 1 cup water
- 2 medium size bananas
- 1/4 tsp bromide plus powder
- 2 tsp light-colored agave syrup

Directions

1. Mash the banana and pour all ingredients into a blender. Blend in for 20 to 30 seconds, incrementing until the mixture is smooth.
2. Dilute with water to your desired thickness.
3. Serve in a cup and add some ice cubes or place in a refrigerator.

Nutrition

Calories: 201, **Protein:** 2.1 g, **Carbs:** 32.4 g, **Fat:** 4.8 g

83. Vegetables Smoothie

10 minutes   0 minutes   1

Ingredients

- 1 carrot
- 1 small beet
- 1 celery stalk
- 1/2 cup raspberries
- 1 cup coconut water
- 1 tsp balsamic vinegar
- Ice (optional)

Directions

1. Blend the carrot, beet, celery, coconut water, raspberries, balsamic vinegar, and ice in a blender (if using). Blend until completely smooth.

Nutrition

Calories: 125, **Fat:** 0.5 g, **Carbs:** 24.8 g, **Protein:** 5.4 g

84. Green Apple Smoothie

10 minutes   0 minutes   1

Ingredients

- 1/2 cup coconut water
- 1 green apple
- 1 cup spinach
- 1/2 cucumber
- 2 tsp raw honey, or maple syrup
- Ice (optional)

Directions

1. Combine the coconut water, apple, spinach, cucumber, honey, and ice in a blender (if using). Blend until completely smooth.

Nutrition

Calories: 226, **Fat:** 4.4 g, **Carbs:** 43.6 g, **Protein:** 2.5 g

85. Cherry Smoothie

10 minutes   0 minutes   1

Ingredients

- 1 cup frozen no-added-sugar pitted cherries
- 1/4 cup raspberries
- 3/4 cup coconut water
- 1 tbsp raw honey or maple syrup
- 1 tsp chia seeds
- 1 tsp hemp seeds
- 6 drops vanilla extract
- Ice (optional)

Directions

1. Blend the cherries, raspberries, coconut water, honey, chia seeds, hemp seeds, vanilla, and ice in a blender until smooth (if using). Blend until completely smooth.

Nutrition

Calories: 304, **Fat:** 11 g, **Carbs:** 42 g, **Protein:** 5.8 g

86. Mango-Thyme Smoothie

10 minutes   0 minutes   1

Ingredients

- 1 cup fresh or frozen mango chunks
- 1/2 cup fresh seedless green grapes
- 1/4 fennel bulb
- 1/2 cup unsweetened almond milk
- 1/2 tsp fresh thyme leaves
- A pinch sea salt
- A pinch of pepper
- Ice (optional)

Directions

1. Blend the mango, grapes, fennel, almond milk, sea salt, thyme leaves, pepper, and ice in a mixer until smooth (if using). Blend until completely smooth.

Nutrition

Calories: 173, **Fat:** 2.3 g, **Carbs:** 35.2 g, **Protein:** 2.7 g

87. Peanut Blackberry Smoothie

 5 minutes   0 minutes   1

Ingredients

- 3/4 cup blackberries
- 1 tbsp peanut butter
- 3/4 cup almond milk
- 1/2 banana peeled
- 2 dates, pitted

Directions

1. In your blender, puree the blackberries with peanut butter, almond milk, banana, and dates. Transfer to a bowl and serve cold.
2. Enjoy!

Nutrition

Calories: 240, **Fat:** 11.1 g, **Carbs:** 28.6 g, **Protein:** 6.8 g

88. Healthy Spinach Smoothie

 5 minutes   0 minutes   1

Ingredients

- 1 1/2 cups fresh spinach
- 1/2 cup ice
- 1 1/2 cups cashew milk
- 1 pear, cored & diced
- 1/4 banana
- 1/2 cup water

Directions

1. Add spinach and remaining ingredients into the blender and blend until smooth and creamy.

Nutrition

Calories: 118, **Fat:** 2.5 g, **Carbs:** 22.1 g, **Protein:** 2.1 g

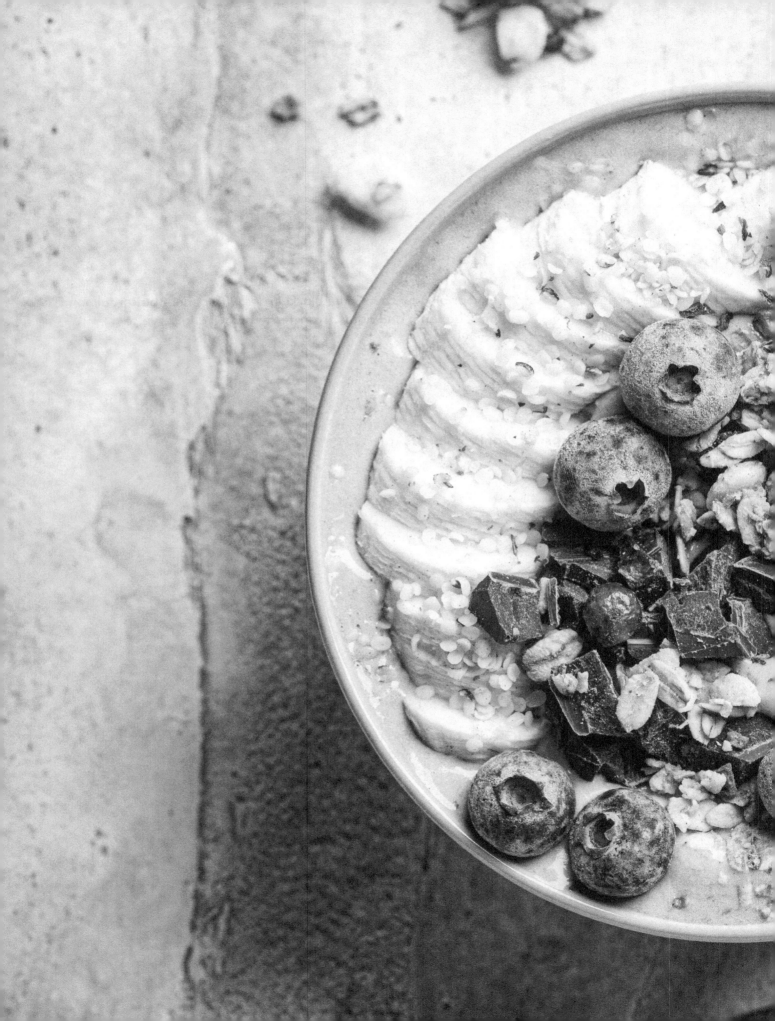

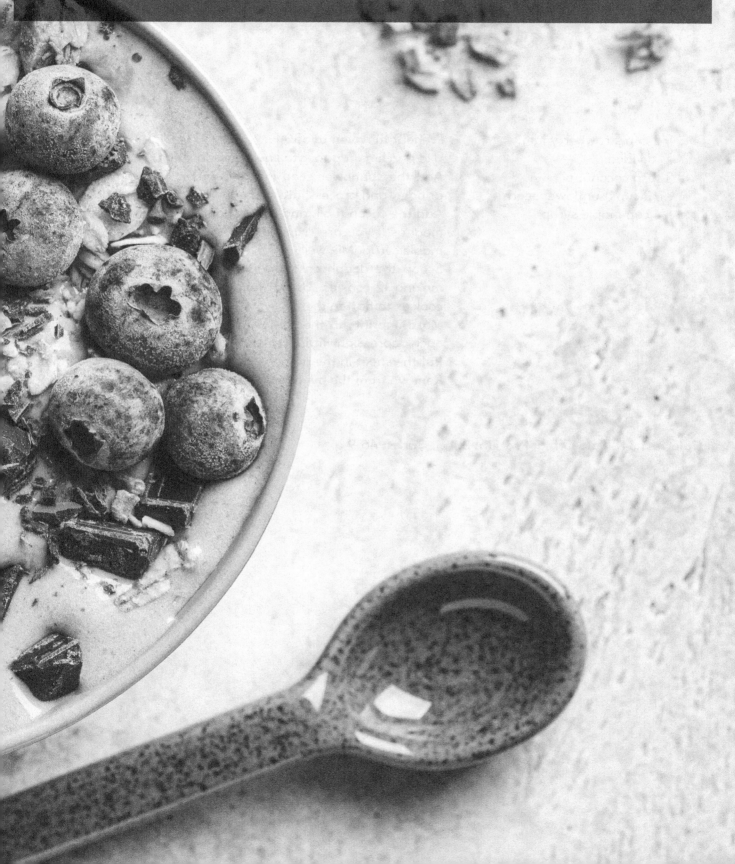

CHAPTER 7
Dessert

89. Strawberry Thumbprint Cookies

15 minutes   15 minutes   5

Ingredients

- 1/2 cup strawberry jam, divided
- 3 tbsp coconut oil
- 1 1/2 cups sunflower seeds
- 1/4 cup maple syrup

Directions

1. Preheat the oven to 350°F.
2. Use parchment paper to line a baking sheet.
3. Add the sunflower seed into a blender, food processor, or spice grinder, and process into a fine meal. Transfer to a large bowl.
4. Add the coconut oil, and use a spoon to mash it into the sunflower meal as if you are crumbling the butter into the flour. Stir in the maple syrup. Mix well.
5. Scoop the dough onto the prepared sheet with 1 tbsp measure, making 12 cookies. Use a wet spoon to gently press down on the cookies to flatten them.
6. Make imprints in the center of each cookie with your thumb. Fill each depression with 2 tsp strawberry jam.
7. Put the sheet in the preheated oven and bake for 12 to 14 minutes.
8. Remove from the oven and let it cool before eating.

Nutrition

Calories: 341, **Fat:** 15.5 g, **Protein:** 3.4 g, **Carbs:** 46.9 g

90. Sweet Banana Pudding

10 minutes   50 minutes   8

Ingredients

- 1/2 cup coconut oil or more
- 1 banana
- 1 organic egg
- 1/2 cup raw honey
- 2 tsp fresh ginger, grated
- 1 tsp pure vanilla extract
- 2 cups almond flour
- A pinch sea salt
- 1 tsp baking soda

Directions

1. Preheat the oven to 350°F.
2. Grease an 8-by-8-inch baking dish with coconut oil, and set aside.
3. In a bowl, beat the coconut oil, banana, egg, honey, ginger, and vanilla with a hand beater until well mixed.
4. Beat together the almond flour, sea salt, and baking soda. Spoon the batter into the dish.
5. Bake for about 50 minutes, until lightly browned.
6. Serve warm.

Nutrition

Calories: 323, **Fat:** 26.1 g, **Protein:** 7.8 g, **Carbs:** 13.7 g

91. Grapefruit Sorbet

10 minutes
+ 4 hours
to freeze

0 minutes

4

Ingredients

For the thyme simple syrup:
- 1/2 cup sugar
- 1/4 cup water
- 1 fresh thyme sprig

For the sorbet:
- Juice of 6 pink grapefruit
- 1/4 cup thyme simple syrup

Directions

1. Combine the sugar, water, and thyme sprig thyme in a small pot. Bring to a boil, remove the heat, and chill until completely chilled. Remove the thyme sprig from the syrup and discard it.
2. Combine the grapefruit juice and thyme simple syrup in a blender and mix until smooth. Freeze for 3 to 4 hours, or until hard, in an airtight container. Serve.

Nutrition

Calories: 195, **Carbs:** 47.2 g, **Protein:** 1.3 g, **Fat:** 0 g

92. Zesty Shortbread Cookies

10 minutes   15 minutes   5

Ingredients

- 1 cup all-purpose flour
- 1/2 cup powdered sugar
- 1/2 cup unsalted butter (cut into 1/2-inch cubes)

Directions

1. Preheat the oven to 375°F. Combine the flour, sugar, and butter in a food processor and process until the dough almost comes together. Take a spoonful of dough and form it into a ball with your hands. Place the dough balls on a baking sheet and continue rolling until all of the dough has been used up.
2. Dip the bottom of a measuring cup in powdered sugar and use the measuring cup to flatten the balls. When the oven is ready, bake for 13 to 15 minutes or until the sides are lightly browned. Allow the cookies to cool on a wire rack. Keep for up to five days in an airtight container.

Nutrition

Calories: 296, **Carbs:** 28.6 g, **Protein:** 3 g, **Fat:** 18.8 g

93. Grape Skillet Galette

 15 minutes   25 minutes   6

+ 2 hours

to chill

Ingredients

For crust:
- 1 cup all-purpose flour
- 1 tbsp sugar
- 4 tbsp cold butter, cut into 1/2-inch cubes
- 1/2 cup Homemade Rice Milk or unsweetened store-bought rice milk

For Galette:
- 1/3 cup sugar
- 1 tbsp cornstarch
- 2 cups halved seedless grapes

Directions

To make the crust:
1. Add the flour and sugar to a food processor and pulse a few times to combine. Pulse in the butter a few times until it resembles a coarse meal. Mix in the rice milk until the dough begins to hold together. Place the dough on a clean surface and roll it out into a flat disc. Refrigerate for 2 hours or overnight after wrapping in plastic wrap.

How to make a Galette:
1. Preheat the oven to 425°F. Combine the sugar and cornstarch in a medium mixing basin. Toss in the grapes to combine. Remove the dough from the wrapper and set it on a floured board. Transfer it to an oven-safe pan and roll it out into a 14-inch circle. Place the grape filling in the middle of the dough and spread it outward, leaving a 2-inch crust border. To partly cover the grapes, fold the dough's edges inward. Cook for 20 to 25 minutes or until golden brown on top. Allow for at least 20 minutes of resting time before serving.

Nutrition

Calories: 244, **Carbs:** 36.6 g, **Protein:** 3.2 g, **Fat:** 9.4 g

94. Baked Apples with Tahini Raisin Filling

10 minutes   35 minutes   6

Ingredients

- 4 ripe apples, cored
- 3/4 cup tahini
- 3 tbsp olive oil
- 1 cup apple juice
- 3 tbsp raisins
- 1/3 cup chopped pecans
- Dash of nutmeg
- Dash of vanilla
- 3/4 cup boiling water

Directions

1. Set the oven to 375°F to preheat. Grease a 9x13-inch baking dish with oil.
2. Place the cored apples in the shallow dish.
3. Mix tahini with half a cup of apple juice in a small bowl.
4. Stir in pecans, raisins, nutmeg, and vanilla. Mix well.
5. Stuff this mixture into the core of the apples.
6. Add some boiling water to the baking dish.
7. Pour the remaining apple juice on top.
8. Bake for 35 minutes until tender.
9. Serve the apples with the remaining juices on top.

Nutrition

Calories: 239, **Fat:** 16.4 g, **Carbs:** 20.2 g, **Protein:** 2.8 g

95. Pistachio and Fruits

5 minutes   7 minutes   1

Ingredients

- 1/2 cup apricots, dried and chopped
- 1/4 cup cranberries, dried
- 1/2 tsp cinnamon
- 1/4 tsp nutmeg, ground
- 1 1/4 cups pistachios, unsalted and roasted
- 2 tsp sugar

Directions

1. Start by heating the oven to a temperature of around 345°F.
2. Using a tray, place the pistachios and bake for 7 minutes. Allow the pistachio to cool afterward.
3. Combine all ingredients in a container.
4. Once everything is combined well, the food is ready to serve.

Nutrition

Calories: 363, **Carbs:** 48.2 g, **Fat:** 15.7 g, **Protein:** 7.3 g

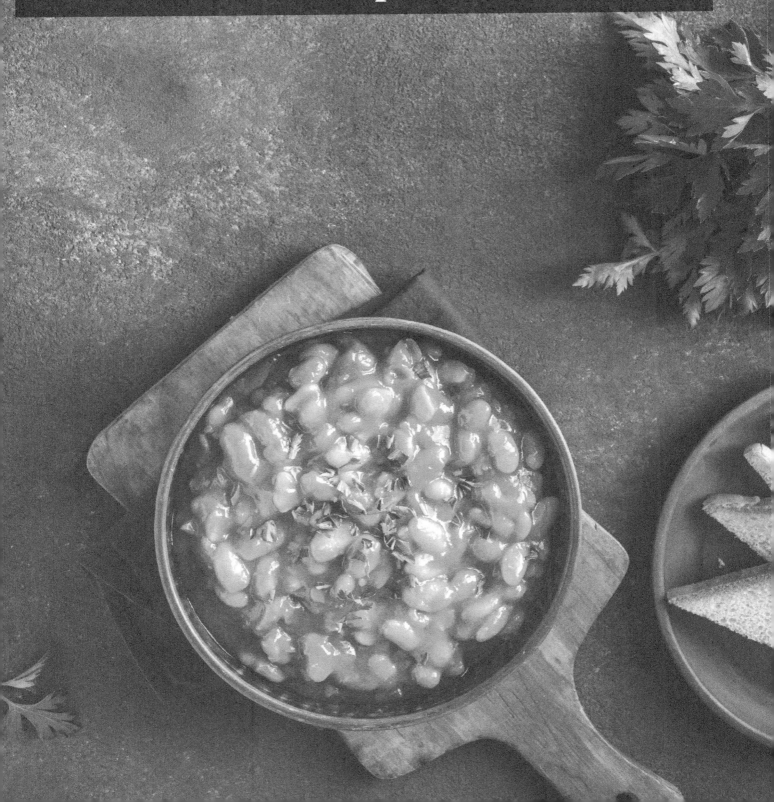

CHAPTER 8
Vegan and Vegetarian Recipes

96. Roasted Broccoli and Cashews

 10 minutes 15 to 20 4

minutes

Ingredients

- 6 cups broccoli florets
- 2 tbsp extra-virgin olive oil
- 1 tsp sea salt
- 1/2 cup toasted cashews
- 1 tbsp coconut aminos

Directions

1. Preheat the oven to 375°F.
2. Combine the broccoli, olive oil, and salt in a large bowl, and toss until the broccoli is coated well.
3. Spread out the broccoli on a baking sheet in a single layer.
4. Roast in the preheated oven for 15 to 20 minutes or until the broccoli is crisp-tender and slightly browned around the edges.
5. Transfer the roasted broccoli to a serving bowl. Allow it to rest for a few minutes until cooled slightly.
6. Add the cashews and coconut aminos to the bowl of broccoli and toss to coat well. Serve immediately.

Nutrition

Calories: 215, **Fat:** 16.3 g, **Protein:** 7.4 g, **Carbs:** 9.8 g

97. Sweet Potatoes and Pea Hash

10 minutes   10 minutes   4

Ingredients

- 2 tbsp coconut oil
- 4 scallions, sliced
- 2 tsp minced fresh ginger
- 1 tsp sea salt
- 2 medium sweet potatoes, roasted in their skins, peeled and chopped
- 2 cups cooked brown rice
- 1 cup frozen peas
- 1 tbsp coconut aminos
- 1/4 cup chopped fresh cilantro, for garnish
- 1/2 cup chopped cashews, for garnish

Directions

1. In a large skillet, melt the coconut oil over medium-high heat.
2. Add the scallions, ginger, curry powder, turmeric, and salt, and stir well. Sauté for 2 minutes until fragrant.
3. Fold in the sweet potatoes, brown rice, peas, and coconut aminos, and sauté for 5 minutes, stirring occasionally.
4. Sprinkle the cilantro and cashews on top for garnish and serve warm.

Nutrition

Calories: 406, **Fat:** 15.5 g, **Protein:** 8.8 g, **Carbs:** 57.8 g

98. Veggie Kabobs

15 minutes   15 minutes   5

Ingredients

For marinade:
- 1 (1-inch) piece fresh ginger, chopped
- 1 tsp ground coriander
- 1/4 cup olive oil
- 1/2 bunch of fresh cilantro
- 1/2 bunch of fresh parsley

For vegetables:
- Olive oil cooking spray
- 2 medium red bell pepper, seeded and cut into 1-inch pieces
- 2 medium zucchinis, cut into 1/3-inch thick round slices
- 1 lb fresh button mushrooms
- 1 large eggplant, quartered lengthwise and cut into 1/2-inch thick slices diagonally

Directions

For the marinade:
1. In a food processor, add all ingredients except for herbs and pulse until well combined
2. Add fresh herbs and pulse until smooth.
3. In a large-sized bowl, add vegetables and marinade and toss to coat well.
4. Refrigerate, covered for about 4 hours.
5. Preheat the grill to medium-low heat.
6. Grease the grill grate with cooking spray.
7. Thread the vegetables onto pre-soaked wooden skewers.
8. Place the skewers onto the grill and cook for about 15 minutes, flipping occasionally.
9. Serve hot.

Nutrition

Calories: 148, **Fat:** 11 g, **Carbs:** 6.7 g, **Protein:** 5.7 g

99. Three Beans Chili

15 minutes   1 hr.   8

Ingredients

- 2 tbsp olive oil
- 1 green bell pepper, seeded and chopped
- 2 celery stalks, chopped
- 1 scallion, chopped
- 1 tsp dried oregano, crushed
- 1 tsp Salt
- 4 cups water
- 16 oz canned cannellini beans drained and rinsed
- 16 oz canned kidney beans, drained and rinsed
- 1/2 of (16 oz) can black beans, drained and rinsed

Directions

1. In a large-sized pan, heat oil over medium heat and cook the bell peppers, celery, and scallion for about 8 to 10 minutes, stirring frequently.
2. Add the oregano, spices, salt, and water and bring to a rolling boil.
3. Simmer for about 20 minutes.
4. Stir in the beans and simmer for about 30 minutes.
5. Serve hot.

Nutrition

Calories: 327, **Fat:** 4.8 g, **Carbs:** 52 g, **Protein:** 19 g

100. Enjoyable Green Lettuce and Bean Medley

10 minutes   4 hours   2

Ingredients

- 3 carrots (sliced)
- 1 cup great Northern beans (dried)
- 1/4 tsp oregano (dried)
- 2 1/2 oz baby green lettuce
- 2 1/2 cups low sodium veggie stock

Directions

1. Combine the beans, carrots, oregano, and stock in Cooker. Stir everything together well. Cook for 4 hours on HIGH with the lid on. Combine the ingredients in a mixing bowl. Allow for an 8-minute rest period after stirring. Serve by dividing the mixture between serving dishes.

Nutrition

Calories: 495, **Carbs:** 80.1 g, **Protein:** 33.2 g, **Fat:** 4.4 g

101. Basil Zucchini Spaghetti

1 hour 10   10 minutes   4

minutes

Ingredients

- 1/3 cup coconut oil (melted)
- 4 zucchinis (cut with a spiralizer)
- 1/4 cup basil (chopped)
- 1/4 cup walnuts (chopped)
- A pinch of sea salt

Directions

1. Mix zucchini spaghetti with salt in a mixing basin, tossing to coat, set aside for 1 hour, drain thoroughly, and place in a bowl. Warm the oil in a pan over medium-high heat, add the zucchini spaghetti, swirl to combine, and cook for 5 minutes. Stir in the basil, and walnuts, and simmer for another 3 minutes. Serve as a side dish by dividing the mixture across plates. Enjoy.

Nutrition

Calories: 238, **Carbs:** 3.5 g, **Protein:** 3.9 g, **Fat:** 23.3 g

102. Healthy, Blistered Beans and Almonds

 10 minutes   20 minutes   2

Ingredients

- 1/2 lb fresh green beans (ends trimmed)
- 1 tbsp olive oil
- 1 tbsp fresh dill (minced)
- 1/8 cup crushed almonds
- 1/8 tsp salt
- 1 tsp salt

Directions

1. Preheat the oven to 400°F. Combine the green beans, olive oil, and salt in a bowl. After that, lay them out on a broadsheet pan. Roast for 10 minutes, then mix well and roast for another 8 to 10 minutes. Please remove it from the oven and continue to whisk in the dill. Serve with crushed almonds and a pinch of sea salt on top.

Nutrition

Calories: 214, **Carbs:** 13 g, **Protein:** 17.2 g, **Fat:** 12.8 g

CHAPTER 9
28-Day Meal Plan

DAYS	BREAKFAST	LUNCH	DINNER	SNACK/DESSERT
1	Steel Cut Oatmeal	Roasted Vegetable Soup	Quick Spinach Salad	Zucchini Hummus
2	Coconut Porridge	Mesmerizing Lentil Soup	Cream of Mushroom Soup	Salmon Canapés
3	Broccoli and Squash Mix	Broccoli Soup	Leeks Soup	Sweet Potato Fries
4	Transition Breakfast Muesli	Cauliflower Soup	Purple Potato Soup	Nuts and Seeds Mix
5	Alkaline Fiber Muesli	Veggie Lunch Salad	Carrot Cucumber Salad	Crispy Baked Kale Chips
6	Banana Date Porridge	Smoked Turkey Salad	Pork Salad	Roasted Vegetables
7	Blueberry Banana Baked Oatmeal	Chopped Greek Salad	Cucumber Soup	Wheat Treats
8	Seedy Breakfast	Cranberry Salad	Tuna and Vegetable Salad	Crispy Roasted Cauliflower
9	Pistachio and Pecan Granola	Summertime Fruit Salad	Cabbage and Scallions Salad	Curry-Spiced Nut Mix with Maple Syrup
10	Walnuts Granola for Breakfast	Cabbage and Almond Salad	Healthy Fruit Salad With Yogurt Cream	Baked Herb Zucchini Chips
11	Baked Apples With Ginger	Seafood Noodles	Duck With Bok Choy	Sweet Potato and Celery Root Mash
12	Pine Nut Pesto with Basil	Oat and Chickpea Dumplings	Pork Chops and Sauce	Spiced Nuts
13	Watermelon Salad	Rosemary lamb bowls	Sauerkraut Soup and Beef	Homemade Guacamole
14	Avocado Smoothie	Rosemary Broiled Shrimp	Turkey Stew	Kale Chips

15	Green Smoothie	Chicken and Pumpkin Stew	Easy Turkey Meatloaf	Strawberry Thumbprint Cookies
16	Pear and Green Tea Smoothie	Tender Stir-Fry Chicken	Thyme Chard-Turkey Burgers	Sweet Banana Pudding
17	Sunshine Smoothie	Tender Coconut Chicken	Vegetarian Pizza With Autumn Toppings	Grapefruit Sorbet
18	Refreshing Apple Smoothie	Mushroom Pork Chops	Mackerel Stew	Zesty Shortbread Cookies
19	Delicious Mango Smoothie	Coconut Zucchini Cream	Tuna Stew	Grape Skillet Galette
20	Raspberry and Chard Smoothie	Split Pea Soup With Coconut	Balsamic Scallops	Strawberry Pie
21	Apple, Berries, and Kale Smoothie	Chicken and Lentil Casserole	Herb Lamb	Baked Apples With Tahini Raisin Filling
22	Banana Alkaline Smoothie	Eggplant Salad	Chicken With Parsley Sauce	Zucchini Hummus
23	Vegetables Smoothie	Cauliflower Rice and Coconut	Healthy, Blistered Beans and Almonds	Salmon Canapés
24	Cherry Smoothie	Summer Vegetable Sauté	Basil Zucchini Spaghetti	Sweet Potato Fries
25	Green Apple Smoothie	Broccoli Blossom	Hot German Cabbage	Nuts and Seeds Mix
26	Mango-Thyme Smoothie	Enjoyable Green Lettuce and Bean Medley	Cauliflower and Dill Mash	Crispy Baked Kale Chips
27	Peanut Blackberry Smoothie	Veggie Kabobs	Three Beans Chili	Roasted Vegetables
28	Healthy Spinach Smoothie	Roasted Broccoli and Cashews	Sweet Potatoes and Pea Hash	Wheat Treats

CHAPTER 10
Shopping List + Cooking Conversion Chart

Making a shopping list is the first step in ensuring that you have everything you need. You must be aware of what you have and what you require. This will prevent you from purchasing unnecessary items and ensure that you only purchase what you truly require. It is also an excellent way to save money. When we don't have a list, we frequently overestimate what we'll need for the month.

Meal planning before going grocery shopping for the week also assists you in purchasing the right items. If you know what you're going to eat, you'll know what ingredients you'll need. This metric is especially useful when purchasing fresh produce. Because these items spoil quickly, purchasing too many is a waste.

With this in mind, let's create a shopping list that will be useful to you. There are things you should always have in your pantry and things you will need to buy every week. Here's an example of what you should get:

- Leafy greens, broccoli, cauliflower, asparagus, carrots, potatoes, peas, beets, sweet potato, butternut squash, and sweet corn are all examples of vegetables. Purchasing frozen vegetables allows you to buy in bulk and use them for a longer time.
- Bananas, apples, pears, melons, apricots, plums, and coconut are examples of fruits. Fruit is always best when it is fresh, so buy it weekly.
- Bulgur, quinoa, brown rice, and rolled oats are examples of whole grains.
- Chicken breast, fish, turkey mince, lentils, and beans are all good sources of protein. You can eat red meat if it is very lean and you don't eat it all the time.
- Herbs and spices—Brazil, oregano, rosemary, thyme, and parsley.

Measurement Conversions

Volume Equivalents (Liquid)

US STANDARD	US STANDARD (OUNCES)	METRIC (APPROXIMATE)
2 tbsp	1 fl. oz.	30 mL
1/4 cup	2 fl. oz.	60 mL
1/2 cup	4 fl. oz.	120 mL
1 cup	8 fl. oz.	240 mL
1 1/2 cups	12 fl. oz.	355 mL
2 cups or 1 pint	16 fl. oz.	475 mL
4 cups or 1 quart	32 fl. oz.	1 L
1 gallon	128 fl. oz.	4 L

Volume Equivalents (Dry)

US STANDARD	METRIC (APPROXIMATE)
1/8 tsp	0.5 mL
1/4 tsp	1 mL
1/2 tsp	2 mL
3/4 tsp	4 mL
1 tsp	5 mL
1 tbsp	15 mL
1/4 cup	59 mL
1/3 cup	79 mL
1/2 cup	118 mL
2/3 cup	156 mL
3/4 cup	177 mL
1 cup	235 mL

2 cups or 1 pint	475 mL
3 cups	700 mL
4 cups or 1 quart	1 L

Oven Temperatures

FAHRENHEIT (F)	CELSIUS (C) (APPROXIMATE)
250°F	120°C
300°F	150°C
325°F	165°C
350°F	180°C
375°F	190°C
400°F	200°C
425°F	220°C
450°F	230°C

Weight Equivalents

US STANDARD	METRIC (APPROXIMATE)
1/2 ounce	15 g
1 ounce	30 g
2 ounces	60 g
4 ounces	115 g
8 ounces	225 g
12 ounces	340 g
16 ounces or 1 pound	455 g

Conclusion

Thank you for making it to the end of this acid reflux cookbook. Acid reflux is a relatively common condition. According to a literature review published in the journal Gut, GERD affects 10 to 20% of the population, and Healthline reports that at least 60% of the population will experience acid reflux within 12 months, with 20 to 30% experiencing weekly symptoms. Although many people believe that GERD is primarily a disease of the elderly, it can affect people of all ages. So, if you suffer from acid reflux, know that you're not alone. The symptoms can range from mild to debilitating, and they can have an impact on many aspects of your life. As you consider changing your diet and lifestyle to help alleviate your symptoms, you may feel overwhelmed. Making significant dietary and lifestyle changes can be stressful for a variety of reasons.

Learning about eating for a specific health condition takes time, and it's difficult to distinguish between good and bad information. There are a lot of people who suffer in silence or ignore the symptoms of acid reflux. Ignoring it is the worst thing you could do. It could lead to more serious issues in the future. It's nothing to be ashamed of.

Making lifestyle changes can help you treat the symptoms of gastroesophageal reflux disease (GERD). To get rid of the symptoms of gastroesophageal reflux disease, you must lose weight if you are overweight or obese. It's also a good idea to avoid drinks and foods that make your symptoms worse two to three hours before bedtime. This GERD cookbook contains a variety of delectable recipes that will not only help you overcome acid reflux but will also keep you healthy for years to come.

Good luck.

THANKS
FOR YOUR PURCHASE!

IF YOU ENJOYED THE BOOK AND WISH TO EXPLORE
FURTHER, I HAVE A SPECIAL SURPRISE IN STORE FOR YOU!
SCAN THE QR CODE BELOW AND DISCOVER EXCLUSIVE
CONTENT AND ADDITIONAL BONUSES THAT I'M SURE WILL
FASCINATE YOU.

I WOULD ALSO BE GRATEFUL IF YOU COULD
LEAVE ME AN HONEST **REVIEW** OF MY WORK.

WITH GRATITUDE,

Lindsey Rush

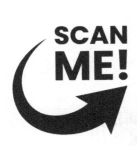

Made in the USA
Las Vegas, NV
20 February 2024